Cardiac Pharmacology

Second Edition

Harilal Nair
DNP, APRN-BC, ANP-C, CCRN, CMC,CSC

APRN WORLD LLC
CALIFORNIA, USA

Publisher's statement

Disclaimer

This book is designed for both beginners and professionals alike,to create better understanding of pharmacologic agents in management of cardiac disorders. This book should not be considered as a substitution to prompt clinical judgment and established medical guidelines for actual patient care. The author and reviewers made tremendous efforts to include most accurate and up to date information in this book. Because of the dynamic nature of modern medicine, the publishers strongly encourage individual learners to identify most updated information from established and reliable sources for day to day patient care.

ISBN-13 978-1-941004-12-8

Library of Congress Control Number - 2018905749

Publisher Information
APRNWORLD LLC
https://aprnworld.com

Printed and published in USA 2018

Preface

Cardiac Pharmacology book is designed for both beginners and professionals as a quick reference for pharmacologic agents used in day-to-day cardiology practice. To provide a simplified and comprehensive view of pharmacologic therapy, we have taken an approach to combine a concise review of basic anatomy and physiology along with pharmacodynamics of various agents. We used simplified explanations whenever possible throughout this book.

Major pharmacologic agent's mechanism of action, interaction and other practical considerations in clinical scenarios are explained in this book. We made a great effort to keep the layout as simple and visually appealing as possible. We used colored graphics and highlights throughout to make the tough topic of pharmacology as interesting as possible for professionals across the age and practice spectrum.

From simple to complex and concrete to abstract ideas, this book is designed as a quick reference and review at bedside. Because of the dynamic nature of pharmacotherapeutics, we strongly advise readers to use updated clinical decision-making tools to make ongoing patient care decision.

We highly appreciate the comments and feedback we received on the previous editions. We, at APRN WORLD, are committed to improve our products and services for serving our clients. Please feel free to drop in your comments through our website HTTP://aprnworld.com. Again, thank you for the ongoing support and encouragement.

Sincerely

Harilal Nair DNP APRN-BC, ANP-C, CCRN, CMC, CSC

Thank God

Table of Contents

1 Basics of Pharmacology

Pharmacology is the biomedical science involving study of drugs and their interaction within the human body. The term 'pharmacology' is derived from Greek language, meaning the **study or knowledge of drugs**. Better understanding of the basic principles of pharmacology is very helpful in evaluating the action, mechanism, interaction and side effects of various pharmacologic agents. Fundamental principles of pharmacology are explained in this chapter.

Pharmacokinetics

Pharmacokinetics refers to the process of movement of a given drug and its metabolic products within the body. This involves **absorption**, **distribution**, **metabolism** and **elimination** of the drug after its administration. In effect, pharmacokinetics is the study of '**how the body affects the drug**'. One of the fundamental principles of pharmacokinetics is that *the concentration of drug at the site of action directly influences the effect of a given drug*. The concentration above and below certain levels can cause undesired or absence of effect at the site of action. In order to understand the factors influencing the concentration of drug at various organs, it is important to identify and analyze the process through which a given drug is absorbed and metabolized in the body. The *range of drug concentration between the minimal effective value and the toxic level* is called **therapeutic window**. Therefore, a drug at its therapeutic window provides the desired outcome with minimum toxic effects. The therapeutic window is always a range rather

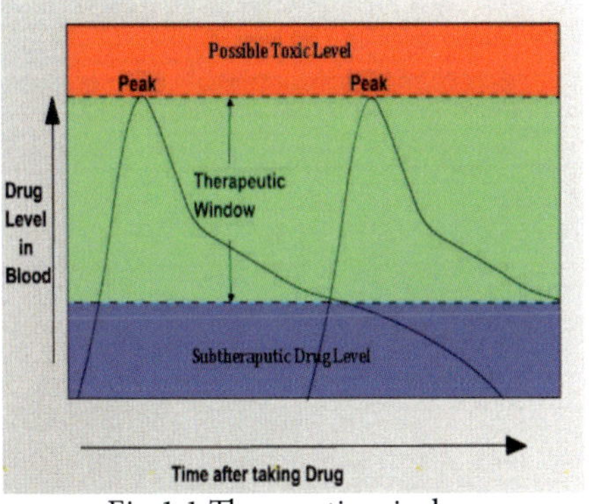

Fig 1.1 Theraputic window

than a definite value because of the unique chemical properties in individual human body.

Factors involving pharmacokinetics of a given drug are

Absorption: Absorption is the process where *a pharmacologic agent passess through physical and physiologic barriers from the site of administration to the systemic circulation*. Common method of drug delivery are **enteral** (oral or rectal route) and **parenteral** (IV, IM or subcutaneous) route. Each one of these administration method possess unique challenges for the pharmacologic agent to reach the systemic circulation and the target organ. **Intravenous (IV) route** is the *most effective and rapid administration method* because the drug is already in the systemic circulation without having to go through multiple physical and chemical barriers. In intramuscular (IM) and subcutaneous (SQ) route, the rate of absorption of the given drug is largely depending on the blood flow to the site of injection and the type of preparation such as oil based or as suspension which delays the process of drug absorption.

Common Mechanisms of Drug Absorption

Diffusion: This is a process by which the chemical *moves from a higher concentration* (from the blood) *to a lower concentration* (to the tissue). It can be simple diffusion or a carrier mediated diffusion. This process *does not require energy expenditure at the cellular level*. The rate of diffusion depends on the strength of the barrier, size of the molecule and the distance that the molecule has to travel. The relationship between these factors and the rate of diffusion is known as **Fick's law** and it states that *the greater the distance and larger the molecule, the slower the diffusion*.

Active transport: This involves movement of the drug from *a lower concentration to a higher concentration with use of energy*. This method is particularly useful in molecules with a positive or negative charge.

Pinocytosis: This process is helpful in transporting fat soluble chemicals across cell membrane. Here, *the cell engulfs the drug particle which is contained in a lipid molecule*. This is a form of active transport.

Box 1.1. Common mechanisms of drug absorption

During enteral administration (oral or rectal route), the drug has to go through multiple chemical and physical barriers such as intestinal mucosa, liver etc. Common mechanisms of drug absorption are shown in the box.

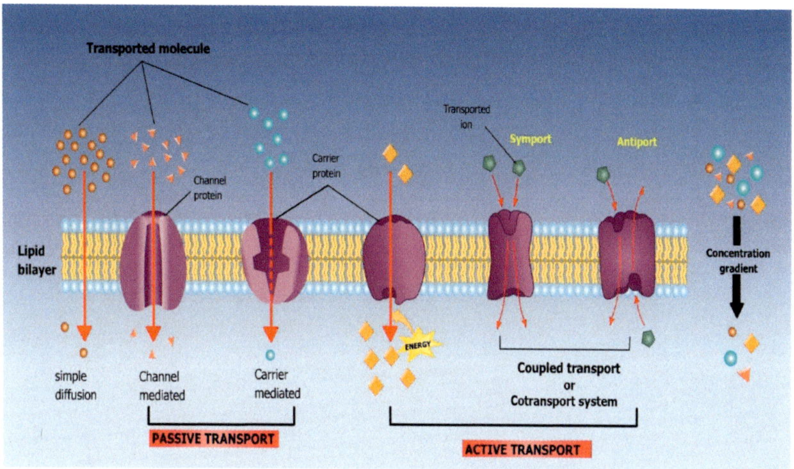

Fig 1.2 Transport of molecules across membranes

An important factor determining the rate of diffusion is the solubility and ionic nature of the drug. For example, lipid soluble drugs can easily penetrate the fatty cells however, water-soluble drugs cannot do the same. This is the reason behind the ability of some of the drugs to pass through physiologic membranes like blood brain barrier. Electrical charge of the drug molecule is another determinant in drug transport as the cells actively regulate number of charged particles to maintain electrical balance. This also affect the absorption of the drugs from acidic environment like the stomach.

Absorption of orally administered drugs mainly happens through the small intestine as the mucosal villi provide a large surface area for the molecules to transport into the bloodstream. *The longer the molecule comes in contact with optimal surface for absorption*, *the greater the drug uptake*. Therefore, factors like intestinal motility as in the case of delayed gastric emptying in presence of high fatty meals or rapid gastric emptying in diarrhea or laxative administration can influence the amount of drug absorption into the systemic circulation.

The drug molecules absorbed from the gastrointestinal

tract goes directly to the liver through portal vein before it reaches into the systemic circulation. Here, *the liver acts as a line of defense by reducing the amount of active drug getting in the systemic circulation*. Certain drugs extensively get metabolized in the liver (**First pass metabolism**) and therefore a *proportionately higher dose has to be administered when given orally compared to intravenous or sublingual route* to achieve same blood concentration.

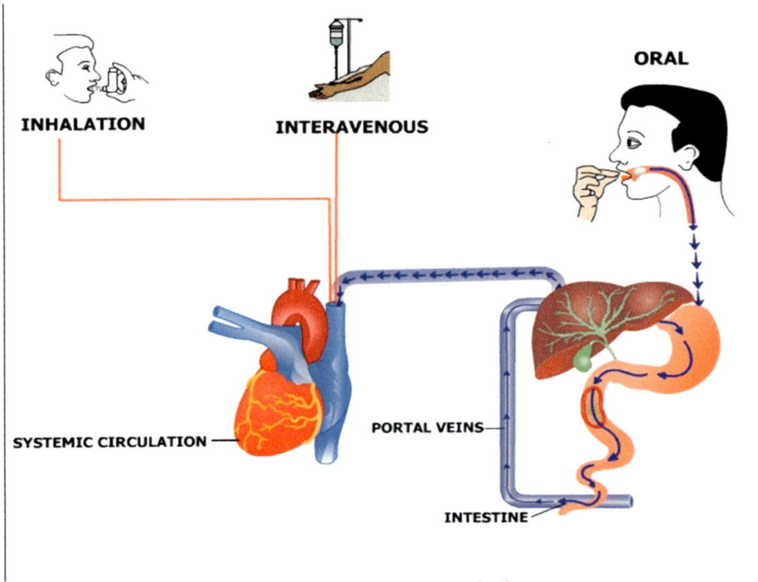

Fig 1.3 First pass metabolism

For example, Morphine has significant first pass metabolism. Therefore, oral dose of Morphine should be three times the intravenous dose to achieve the same therapeutic effect. Hence, a person receiving 10 mg of intravenous morphine over 24 hours period should have 30 mg of oral morphine preparation in the same time frame in order to get the desired effect. This knowledge is very important in calculating the dosage of drugs with extensive first pass metabolism such as Lidocaine, Imipramine, Nitroglycerin, Propranolol, Quinidine, Coumadin, Theophylline etc.

Bioavailability is the *amount of drug that reaches into the systemic circulation after its first pass metabolism*. Bioavailability can also be influenced by the **solubility of the drug**, **interaction of drug with gastric pH** etc. All these factors can be altered by adding inert ingredients or protective coatings on capsules or tablets. This is the mechanism behind extended-release or sustained release forms of various medications. *Because of the absence of first pass metabolism, majority of intravenously administered drugs have 100% bioavailability*. This is the reason why Lidocaine, which has extensive first pass metabolism in the liver, is not administered orally and is always given in the intravenous route. **Bioavailability** of the drug can also be influenced by **genetic factors** and coexisting disease conditions ike **liver dysfunction**. Therefore, in day-to-day clinical practice it is very important to identify these factors to prevent sub-therapeutic dosing or toxic side-effects from drugs with a narrow therapeutic window.

Distribution

After absorbed in to the systemic circulation, *the drugs get distributed throughout the body depending on the cardiac output*, *regional blood flow*, *body composition* and *binding properties* of the given chemical. Transport of the drug in plasma can either be bound to the plasma proteins or as free drug molecules. *Acidic drugs attached with albumin* whereas *basic drugs bind with plasma lipoproteins* for the purpose of transport. The binding between transport particles and the drug molecule is reversible in such a way that when the free drug is either eliminated or metabolized, the bound drug can be unchained to maintain the equilibrium. Therefore, *the protein-bound part acts as a reservoir of the drug*.

When administering together, some drugs compete each other for plasma protein molecules and the drug with strongest affinity towards the carrier molecule gets attached. This leaves the other drug unbound to the carrier molecule and essentially results in a transient increase in the concentration of free drug in systemic circulation.

The affinity of the drug towards the carrier particle depends on the concentration of the drug and the carrier. For example, in patients with low serum album, there is less number of carrier particles available for drug transport, resulting in unusually large amount of free drug in the systemic circulation. The proportion of the drug bound to the protein is unavailable for receptor site stimulation. Therefore, *the effect of a particular drug is determined by the amount of free drug in the plasma*. This information is very important in patients with low serum albumin (**hypoalbuminemia**), which is one of the common plasma proteins for drug transport. These patients will have a high amount of free drug in the plasma and hence chance of toxic side-effects. Clinical conditions with low amount of plasma proteins like nephrotic syndrome, burns and liver disease demand dosage adjustments.

Volume of distribution of a drug depends on whether the drug is lipid soluble or water-soluble. *Water-soluble drugs predominantly stay in the circulatory system and therefore have a relatively low volume of distribution*. Hence, majority of water soluble drugs once administered are available either for desired action or for excretion. However, lipid soluble drugs penetrate through various physiologic barriers in the body and start storing in bones, muscles and other compartments. Since the portion of the drug trapped in these compartments are not readily available for metabolism or excretion, the effect can be prolonged (e.g. Amiodarone).

Metabolism

The Primary Purpose of metabolism is *to facilitate excretion of the drug from the body*. The drug becomes more water-soluble after metabolism. Increased water solubility helps in excretion of drug through the kidney. Even though most of the drugs become inactive after metabolism, some of them become active only after the initial metabolic process. These drugs are called **pro-drugs**. *Majority of drug metabolism happens in the liver* because of the abundance of hepatic enzyme. The process of hepatic metabolism involves two phases as described below.

Oxidation (**Phase1**): During this process, an oxygen atom is attached to the chemical molecule to make it more water-soluble. This oxidative process is catalyzed by the group of enzymes called **Cytochrome P450** (**CYP 450**). Because of the lipid solubility, most of the lipid soluble drugs pass through CYP 450 for hepatic metabolism. When used together, some of the drugs can cause production of more CYP 450 enzymes and thereby accelerate metabolism of the other drug, known as **CYP 450 enzymes inducers**. This results in decreasing the availability of free drug in the circulation. On the other hand, some drugs can suppress the production of CYP450 enzymes and thereby slowing down the metabolism of the other drug. This mechanism essentially creates a higher concentration of the second drug in the blood. These drugs are known as **CYP 450 enzyme inhibitors**.

Drug to drug interaction based on CYP 450 enzyme system

is very important especially when administering more than one medicine at a time. Knowledge of potential interactions help to avoid possibility of sub therapeutic response or toxic reaction because of enzyme inhibition or induction.

Conjugation (**Phase2**): In this process, another molecule is added to the product from previous steps that enhances water solubility and thereby excretion of the given drug.

CYP 450 System

Cytochrome P450 is a large family of hepatic oxidative enzymes that catalyze drug metabolism. Majority of the drugs are metabolized through four types of Cytochrome P450 systems **CYP3A4** (50%), **CYP2D6** (25%) **CYP2C9** (20%) and **CYP1A2** (5%). There are some other systems like **CYP2C19** also involved in metabolism of some of the common cardiac drugs. Even though there are specific genes encoding each CYP450 enzymes, genetic variation in the form of **polymorphism** exist between individuals.

> Absence of specific CYP 450 system enzyme can interfere with metabolism of certain drugs in deficient individuals. For example, Codeine is a pro-drug that metabolizes through CYP2D6 enzyme pathway to become Morphine, which is the active metabolite. Therefore, Codeine can be ineffective in individuals who are deficient in this enzyme. Patients who are taking large amount of Codeine without significant clinical response need to be evaluated for this possibility.

This polymorphic variations result in the same enzyme with three different functional potential known as **ultra-rapid metabolizers**, **extensive metabolizers** and **poor metabolizers**. Since the gene polymorphism is linked to the ethnic backgrounds of individuals, metabolism of certain drugs can vary considerably from person to person with same physical characteristics but of different ethnic origin. The functional difference of these oxidative enzymes play a major role in drug toxicity, drug nonresponsiveness etc.

One of the much-publicized examples for genetic variation of CYP450 system is the case of **Clopidogrel** and **CYP2C19** alleles. It is well documented through a number of clinical research studies that there are a large number of individuals who are nonresponders to Clopidogrel because of the polymorphism of gene CYP2C19

Common Drugs Metabolized by CYP 450 Systems	
CYP3A4	Amiodarone, Dihydropyridine calcium channel blockers (e.g. Amlodipine, Nifedipine) and Non-dihydropyridines (Verapamil and Diltiazem), Coumadin, Lidocaine, Quinidine, Statins group, Sildenafil , Clarithromycin, Erythromycin, oral contraceptives
CYP2D6	Beta-Blockers, Codeine, Propafenone, Mexiletine, Fluoxetine
CYP2C9	Ibuprofen, Coumadin, Losartan, Irbesartan
CYP2C19	Clopidogrel, Omeprazole, Phenytoin, Indomethiacin, Diazepam
CYP1A2	Acetaminophen, Caffeine, Nicotine, Theophylline, Cimatidine, Ciprofloxacin

Box 1.2.Common drugs metabolized by CYP450 systems

causing poor metabolism of the drug. The core problem in the case of Clopidogrel is that *Clopidogrel is a pro-drug that needs to be metabolized in order to become active and cause platelet inhibition*. If the metabolism of pro-drug is interfered with this genetic variation, the amount of active drug available will be much lower than expected, leading to poor therapeutic effect. However, because of the lack of sufficient evidence routine testing for genetic variation is not yet recommended.

Excretion

Even though the elimination of a given drug can be through various organs like lower GI tract, liver, skin etc., the *primary organ for drug excretion is the kidney*. After hepatic metabolism of the drug, the metabolites get filtered through the glomerular filtration system in the kidney. Depending on the chemical nature of the drug, it passes through proximal and distal tubules and loop of Henle where the drug exerts local effect as in the case of diuretics. Thereafter the drug either gets eliminated through urine or reabsorbed back in to the circulation.

Kidneys excrete water-soluble forms of drugs through glomerular filtration, tubular secretion and tubular reabsorption. During **glomerular filtration**, drugs move across glomerular membrane through passive diffusion depending on the molecular size, protein binding etc. During **tubular secretion**, the drugs are **actively transported** from the blood to the urine. Since it is an active process involving transport systems, *multiple drugs competing for the same transport system can affect the rate of excretion of one another*. Most of the lipid soluble drugs are reabsorbed at the distal convoluted tubules. **pH of the urine** has a major influence in tubular reabsorption process. Drugs that are ionized in to weak acids (pH less than 7) get excreted in urine with alkaline pH and drugs with alkaline nature (pH greater than 7) are excreted in acidic urine. *Ionization gives capacity for the drug to be soluble in water and there by facilitate excretion*.

In order to understand the patient's kidney function, a surrogate marker called **Creatinine clearance** is used instead of glomerular filtration rate (GFR). **Creatinine** is a product of muscle breakdown and is continually excreted through glomerular filtration without significant tubular secretion or reabsorption. Therefore, ability of the kidney to excrete Creatinine is a good measure of patient's kidney function. *Creatinine clearance of less than 50 ml/min represents severely impaired kidney function* and therefore dosage adjustments to be made for drugs having major renal excretion pathway.

For example, **Enoxaparin,** a low molecular weight heparin with major renal excretion pathway, has a recomended dose of 1mg/kg Q12hour for patients with Non ST Segment elevation myocardial infarction (NSTEMI). Similar patients with Creatinine clearance less than 30ml/ min only require half of the recomended dose for therapeutic effect.

Some drugs are excreted by the liver in to the gall bladder in conjugated forms through bile and are subsequently excreted in to the GI tract. Because of the effect of intestinal bacteria, these drugs can be freed from their conjugation. The resultant free drug may absorb back to the systemic circulation. This process is called **enterohepatic recirculation**. Manufactures take the effect of enterohepatic reabsorption in to consideration while formulating the drug dosages in order to avoid drug toxicity.

However, in the absence of these gut bacteria and the enzymes as in the case of concomitant use of antibiotics, enterohepatic reabsorption may not be effective, leading to lower than expected concentration of the drug in the blood. For example,

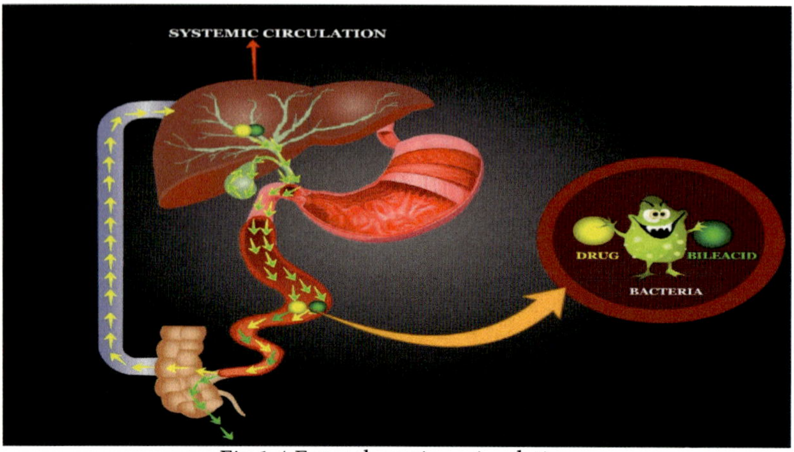

Fig 1.4 Enterohepatic recirculation

while using oral contraceptives and antibiotics together, because of the significant reduction in enterohepatic reabsorption, the therapeutic blood level of oral contraceptives may not be attained. This may results in treatment failure of oral contraceptives. Enterohepatic recirculation is also responsible for delay in clearance of drugs from the body and thereby prolonged effect.

Half-life

The half-life of a drug is defined as *the time required for plasma concentrations to be decreased by one half*. The half-life of a given drug depends on factors like the nature of the drug, renal and hepatic function etc. *With every half-life*, *50% of the remaining amount of drug is excreted* from the body. For example, if the half-life of a given drug is 8 hours, that is the time taken for half of the drug to be excreted from the body. So if the plasma concentration is 100mg/L at the beginning, after one half-life (i.e.8 hrs), the concentration will become 50 mg/L. After second half-life (i.e. 16 hrs), 50% of the remaining drug is excreted and therefore the concentration

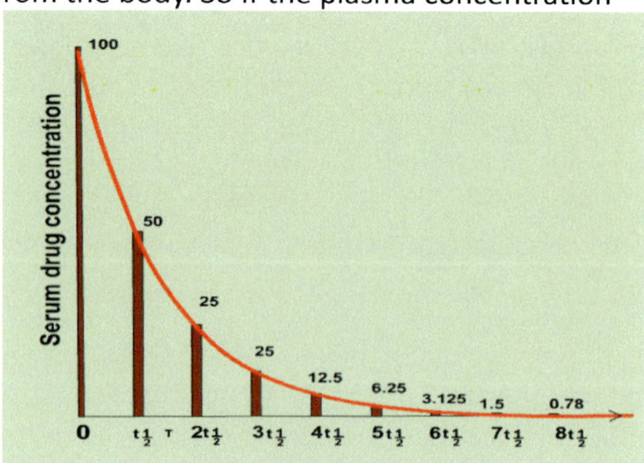

Fig 1.5 Half life of a drug

becomes 25mg/L. When this process continues, the concentration becomes 12.5 mg/L and 6.25 mg/L after third (24 hrs) and forth (36 hrs) half lives respectively.

It is interesting to see that after three half-lives, the effective serum level of the drug is around 10% of its original concentration. *After five half-lives, the amount of drug remains in the system is practically negligible*. At that concentration, the drug may not be able to create any pharmacologic effects in the body. This information is very useful in identifying the timing for administration of next dose in order to maintain a therapeutic blood level. It is also helpful in drug toxicity situations to understand when the patient will have a safer blood level of the overdosed drug. Since the half life is also influenced by kidney and liver function, it is important to adjust the dosage of drugs in patients with these organ dysfunction.

It is important to remember that half life is not the absolute entity determine the availability of a drug in the body after its administration. A myriad of factors like volume of distribution, lipid solubility, affinity for proteins etc. are also strongly influence the performance of a drug in the body. For example, Amiodarone which has a large volume of distribution; accumulates in the body tissues and therefore the effect can extend up to 50 days after discontinuation of the drug.

Pharmacodynamics

Pharmacodynamics is essentially the study of the effects of drugs in the body. This branch of pharmacology deals with *the interaction between the drug and the chemical receptors within the body*. Pharmacodynamics also measures the potency and efficacy of a given drug. In order to understand the effect of drugs at various target organs through drug- receptor interaction, consider *the receptors as the lock and the drugs as a key to operate them*. Depending on the type of the drugs, they can facilitate or inhibit physiologic functions. The drugs that facilitate chemical processes by combining with receptor sites are called **agonist** and those who inhibit the processes are known as **antagonist** or **blockers**. One of the fundamental principles of pharmacology is that the *therapeutic effect of drug is proportional to the amount of drug available at the site of action*. Based on this principle, when there are more drug molecules present at the site of action, they combine with more receptor sites to accelerate the biologic process. However, there are only a fixed number of receptor sites available for action and therefore increasing the concentration of drug beyond a particular level does not elicit any more speed in the biologic function. This point where all the receptor sites are occupied at the site of action is called **saturation**.

Similarly, if the receptors are stimulated by the drug at the maximal capacity for a long time, the receptors become less sensitive to the drug by the process known as **down regulation** or **desensitization**. This is a natural mechanism to prevent overstimulation from any given chemical. This down regulation of receptors cause **tachyphylaxis** in clinical practice. One of the examples is that after giving transdermal preparation of Nitroglycerine for long duration, patients do not develop any desired effect unless there are drug free intervals in the administration schedule. Therefore, physicians usually prescribe these patches to be worn only for certain number of hours during a 24 hr period. Severe down regulation of receptor activity may create a lack of responsiveness to the drug called **refractoriness**.

Antagonist or inhibitory drug receptor interaction can create unique challenges in clinical practice. If a group of receptors are down regulated or antagonized or inhibited for a long duration, sudden withdrawal of such drugs cause over stimulation of the receptor from the natural agonist in the body. For example, rapid withdrawal of centrally acting antihypertensive such as Clonidine may cause 'rebound hypertension'. Therefore, these drugs are tapered down in their doses before complete withdrawal in order for the receptors to get back to normal sensitivity.

The drugs can create reversible or irreversible bonds with a receptors site or the enzymes in the metabolic pathway. If the drug molecules are reversibly attached to the receptor sites, they are called **competitive agonist** or **antagonist**. If there are two drugs compete for the same receptor site like in the case of hepatic drug metabolism through CYP450 pathway, the drug with higher concentration or chemical affinity can get attached to the receptor site and block the other one's action. This effect is seen in concomitant administration of proton pump inhibitors (e.g. Omeprazole, Esomeprazole) and antiplatelet Clopidogrel (Plavix).

Here, because of the competition for the same enzyme receptor site, Clopidogrel get blocked from receptors by the proton pump inhibitors.

Food Drug Interaction

Food products can affect the absorption, metabolism, and excretion of various drugs in the body. As far as the absorption of drugs is concerned, food items can combine with the drugs to make them ineffective (e.g. presence of milk in the stomach can interfere with absorption of Ciprofloxacin) or act as a physical barrier that prevents the drug from reaching the mucosal surface of the GI tract. *In presence of a high fatty meal*, *the absorption of lipophilic drugs are generally enhanced*. Some food items can inhibit the therapeutic response of a given drug as in the case of green leafy vegetables and Coumadin. In this situation, *eating significantly large amount of green leafy vegetables which are high in vitamin K will decrease INR below predicted levels by negating Coumadin effect*. Grapefruit juice can affect the metabolism of many drugs by inhibiting CYP3A4 enzyme system. *Dihydropyridine calcium channel blockers such as Amlodipine, Nifedipine etc. are known to have significant interaction with grapefruit juice* and therefore should not be given in combination.

Another major and well known food drug interaction is between Tyramine containing food and Monoamine oxidase inhibitor (MAOI), which is an antidepressant. Tyramine is an amino acid with sympathomimetic properties (stimulating sympathetic nervous system causing flight-fight response). Monoamine oxidase is the enzyme that helps in degradation of Tyramine. In presence of MAOI drugs, the degradation process of Tyramine is blocked. The resulting accumulation of Tyramine creates sympathetic overdrive leading to **hypertensive crisis**. Therefore, it is advisable to avoid eating food items with high amount of Tyramine such as fermented foods, chocolate, coffee, wine etc. while taking MAOI drugs.

Adverse Drug Reactions

One of the fundamental principles of pharmacology is that *all drugs are poison unless used in appropriate amounts*. Even with therapeutic dosages, these chemicals have a tendency to develop untoward reactions. **Adverse drug reactions** (**ADR**) are the *symptoms that are uncomfortable but tolerable for the patient.*

At the same time, anaphylactic reactions are those situations *demanding immediate termination of therapy because of life threatening consequences*.

Adverse drug reactions are classified into two main categories as described below.

Classification of Hypersensitivity Reactions

Type I reaction (**Immediate hypersensitivity reaction**): This is an Immunoglobulin E (IgE) mediated reaction that causes release of histamine, prostaglandins and leukotrines; leading to symptoms of urticaria, bronchospasm, angioedema or anaphylactic shock. These symptoms can develop within a time period of 30 min to 12 hours after exposure to the drug.

Type II hypersensitivity reaction (**Cytotoxic hypersensitivity**): This Is an immunoglobulin G or M (IgG or IgM) mediated reaction leading to neutropenia, hemolysis, thrombocytopenia etc. The reaction time can be from minutes to hours.

Type III hypersensitivity (**Immune complex hypersensitivity**): This IgM and IgG mediated reaction can cause serum sickness, fever, joint and muscle pain and lymphadenopathy. These symptoms are usually developed from 8 hrs to 3 wks

Type IV allergic reactions (**Cell mediated or Delayed hypersensitivity**): These type of reactions can take 2-3 days for development and are characterized by contact dermatitis or fixed drug eruptions. One classic example for this type of hypersensitivity reaction is the Tuberculin skin testing (Mantoux testing) or PPD.

Type V allergic reaction (**Autoimmune reaction**): The pathogenesis of this group of hypersensitivity is not exactly identified. Example for type V allergic reactions is 'lupus like disease' when exposed to Amiodarone, Procainamide, Phenytoin etc.

Box 1.3.Classification of hypersensitivity reactions

Type A adverse drug reactions

These are the most common type of adverse drug reaction that constitutes 70 to 80% of reported events. The *symptoms are somewhat predictable and dose-dependent and are related to the given drug's pharmacologic action*. These are better known as side effects. Incidents of hypotension while using antihypertensives, hypoglycemia from use of diabetic medication etc. are some common examples for **type A adverse reactions**. This type of adverse reactions are usually caused either by higher doses of the drug or factors affecting absorption, metabolism or elimination of the drug.

Type B adverse reactions

This type of adverse reactions are *more serious and requires discontinuation of the drug*. Common examples are anaphylactic reactions, urticaria, serum sickness, hemolytic anemia etc. These reactions are unexpected and unavoidable. Drug allergy can be classified based on the timing of symptom onset and type of reaction as described in box 1.3.

Drug Safety During Pregnancy

Many of the pharmacologic agents possess significant maternal and fetal risk (teratogenicity) if used during pregnancy.

Pregnancy Risk Rating for Drugs by FDA

Category	Definition	Cardiovascular drugs
Category A	Controlled human studies show no risk (Safest)	No cardiovascular drugs in this category.
Category B	No evidence of risk in humans (relatively safe)	• Methyldopa • UFH, LMWH • Sotalol (Only in 1st trimester) • Labetalol • Torsemide
Category C	Risk cannot be ruled out (Use with caution)	• Clopidogrel, Ticlopidine • Digoxin • Lidocaine, Amiodarone • Hydralazine, Clonidine, • Metoprolol, Propranolol • Furosemide • Niacin, Gemfibrozil
Category D	positive evidence of risk (Use with extreme caution)	• ACE inhibitors, ARB, Direct Renin inhibitor • Spironolactone • Most of the beta-blockers (especially second and third trimester)
Category X	Animal or human studies have shown risk to the fetus and their risk outweighs benefit. (Contraindicated in pregnancy).	• Statins • Coumadin (except for patients with mechanical valve-category D)

UHF-Unfractionated heparin; **LMWH**-Low Molecular Weight heparin; **ACE**- Angiotensin Converting Enzyme Inhibitors; **ARB**- Angiotensin Receptor Blockers

Table 1.1. Pregnancy risk rating for drugs by FDA

Some of them are contraindicated during the entire pregnancy however, many drugs can be given safely during certain trimesters. Commonly used cardiovascular drugs and their pregnancy classification are described in table 1.1.

Points to remember!!!

- The term 'pharmacology' is derived from Greek language and it means the **study or knowledge of drugs**.
- Pharmacokinetics refers to the process of movement of a given drug and its metabolic products within the body.
- Pharmacokinetics involves **absorption**, **distribution**, **metabolism** and **elimination** of the drug after its administration.
- The concentration of drug at the site of action directly influences the effect of a given drug.
- The range of drug concentration between the minimal effective value and the toxic level is called **therapeutic window**
- Absorption is the process where a pharmacologic agent passes through physical and physiologic barriers from the site of administration to the systemic circulation.
- The longer the molecule comes in contact with optimal surface for absorption, the greater the drug uptake.
- Certain drugs get extensively metabolized in the liver (**First pass metabolism**) and therefore a *proportionately higher dose has to be administered when given orally, compared to intravenous or sublingual route.*
- **Bioavailability** is the *amount of drug that reaches into the systemic circulation after its first pass metabolism.*
- *Because of the absence of the first pass metabolism, majority of intravenously administered drugs have 100% bioavailability.*
- **Bioavailability** of the drug can also be influenced by **genetic factors** as well as coexisting disease conditions such as **liver dysfunction**.
- *Acidic drugs attached with albumin* whereas *basic drugs bind with plasma lipoproteins* for the purpose of transport.
- *The effect of a particular drug is determined by the amount of free drug in the plasma.*

- **Volume of distribution** of a drug depends on whether the drug is lipid soluble or water-soluble.
- *Water-soluble drugs predominantly stay in the circulatory system and therefore have a relatively low volume of distribution.*
- The Primary Purpose of metabolism is *to facilitate excretion of the drug from the body.*
- Kidneys excrete the water-soluble forms of drugs through glomerular filtration, tubular secretion and tubular reabsorption.
- Multiple drugs competing for the same transport system can affect the rate of excretion of one another.
- Ability of the kidney to excrete Creatinine is a good measure of patient's kidney function.
- Creatinine clearance of less than 50 ml/min represents severely impaired kidney function.
- Enterohepatic recirculation can cause delay in clearance of drugs from the body and thereby prolonged effect.
- The half-life of a drug is defined as *the time required for plasma concentrations to be decreased by one half.*
- *With every half-life, 50% of the remaining amount of drug is excreted* from the body.
- *After five half-lives, the amount of drug remains in the system is practically negligible.*
- Pharmacodynamics is the study of *the interaction between the drug and the chemical receptors within the body.*
- The drugs that facilitate chemical process by combining with receptor sites are called **agonist** and those who inhibit the process are known as **antagonist** or **blockers**.
- The point where all the receptor sites are occupied at the site of action is called **saturation**.
- If the receptors are stimulated by the drug at their maximal capacity for a long time, the receptors become less sensitive to the drug by the process known as **down regulation** or **desensitization**.
- Severe down regulation of receptor activity may create a lack of responsiveness to the drug called **refractoriness**.

- If the drug molecules are reversibly attached to the receptor sites, they are called **competitive agonist** or **antagonist**.
- Cytochrome P450 is a large family of hepatic oxidative enzymes that catalyze drug metabolism.
- The polymorphic variations within CYP450 enzymes result in the same enzyme with three different functional potential such as **ultra-rapid metabolizers**, **extensive metabolizers** and **poor metabolizers**.
- *In presence of a high fatty meal, the absorption of lipophilic drugs is generally enhanced.*
- Grapefruit juice can affect the metabolism of many drugs by inhibiting CYP3A4 enzyme system.
- **Adverse drug reaction** (**ADR**) are the *symptoms that are uncomfortable but tolerable for the patient*
- **Anaphylactic reactions** are those situations *demanding immediate termination of therapy because of life threatening consequences.*
- **Type A adverse drug reactions** has *symptoms somewhat predictable and dose-dependent and are related to the given drug's pharmacologic action*. They are also known as 'side effects'.
- **Type B adverse reactions** are *more serious and requires discontinuation of the drug like in the case of* anaphylactic reactions

2 Alpha Receptor Mediated Agents

Autonomic nervous system has a major role in maintaining homeostasis of many organs in the body. This is achieved by maintaining a balance between counteracting forces from two component of autonomic nervous system called **sympathetic** and **parasympathetic nervous systems**. These two autonomic nervous pathways have their own effect on various organs. In general, *sympathetic nervous system helps with excitation and parasympathetic dealt with inhibition or down regulation of various functions*. **Norepinephrine** is the major neurotransmitter involved with sympathetic nervous system whereas, **Acetylcholine** occupies a prominent role in parasympathetic control. Sympathetic nervous system is also called **Adrenergic nervous system** and parasympathetic is known as **Cholinergic nervous system**.

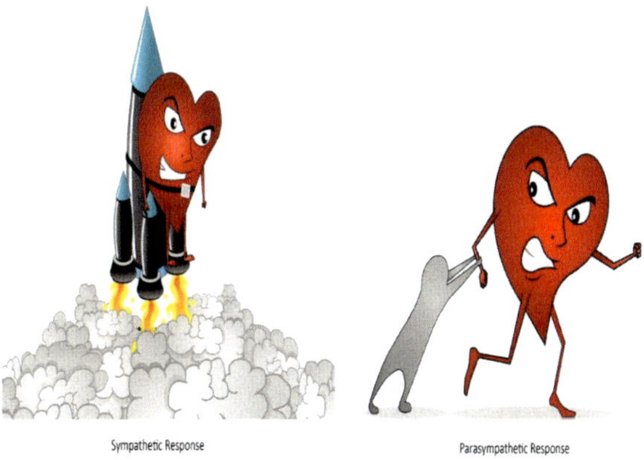

Fig 2.1 Autonomic nervous system influence

Adrenergic Agents

These agents *facilitate sympathetic nervous system activity* by combining with sympathetic receptors such as **Alpha-1**, **Alpha-2**, **Beta -1**and **Beta-2** receptors. Among these, Alpha-1 agonist agents are described in chapter 9 along with ionotropics and vasopressors. Alpha 1 antagonists, Alpha 2 agonists and antagonists are discussed in this chapter. Common examples of various agents with their receptor specificity are shown in the table.

Sympathetic Nervous System Receptors			
Receptor type	**Action**	**Agonist**	**Antagonists**
Alpha 1 receptors	• Smooth muscle contraction • vasoconstriction the skin, mucosa and kidney • GI and bladder sphincter contraction • Facilitate sodium reabsorption from kidney • Increase secretion from sweat glands	Norepinephrine Phenylephrine	Doxazosin Prazosin Terazosin
Alpha-2 receptors	• Smooth muscle relaxation • Platelet activation	Clonidine Guanabenz Guanfacine	Phentolamine (largely nonselective)
Beta-1receptors	• Positive chronotropic (increase heart rate), dromotropic (increasing conduction velocity) and ionotropic (increasing contractility) effect in the heart • increasing Renin secretion	Dobutamine Norepinephrine Isoproterenol	Metoprolol Atenolol Propranolol
Beta-2 receptors	• Smooth muscle relaxation of bronchi and GI tract	Albuterol Isoproterenol Levalbuterol	Propranolol Timolol

Table 2.1 Drugs function through Sympathetic nervous system receptors

Alpha-1 Adrenergic Antagonists

Alpha-1 adrenergic antagonists *selectively block Alpha-1 receptors in the vascular smooth muscle* and thereby reduce peripheral vascular resistance. This reduction in peripheral vascular resistance leads to vasodilation and subsequent lowering of blood pressure. Since these agents *cause reduction in both arterial and venous vascular tone irrespective of the position of the patient*, they cause significant orthostatic hypotension. This made them less favorable for treatment of essential hypertension. However, because of the effect on smooth muscle especially at the bladder neck, many of these agents are used for treatment of Benign Prostatic Hypertrophy (**BPH**). Common agents in this category are shown in the table.

The mechanism by which alpha-1 receptor antagonists reduce symptoms of benign prostatic hypertrophy is that the

Drug	Action	Use
Prazosin (Minipress®)	Selective alpha-1 receptor blockade	Treatment of hypertension and BPH
Doxazosin (Cardura®)	Selective alpha-1 receptor blockade	Treatment of hypertension and BPH
Terazosin (Hytrin®)	Selective alpha-1 receptor blockade	Treatment of hypertension and BPH
Tamsulosin (Flomax®)	Selective alpha-1 receptor blockade	Treatment of only BPH
Alfuzosin (Uroxatral®)	Selective alpha-1 receptor blockade	Treatment of only BPH
Phenoxybenzamine (Dibenzyline®)	Irreversibly block both alpha-1 and alpha-2 receptors	Used for treatment of pheochromocytoma

Table 2.2 Alpha-1 adrenergic blockers

prostate gland and the bladder neck contains large amount of alpha-1 receptors compared to the bladder wall. *Blockade of these alpha-1 receptors cause relaxation of the muscles selectively at prostate gland and bladder neck* without affecting bladder contractility. This helps in relieving obstruction for urine outflow. These drugs are well absorbed through oral intake and are extensively metabolized at liver and excreted through feces and urine.

> Alpha-1 adrenergic antagonists can cause significant orthostatic hypotension especially with first dose or restarting medication after interrupting treatment for a number of days. This effect is intensified if the patient is taking other antihypertensive medications especially vasodilators such as nitrates, PDE-5 inhibitors (Viagra, Cialis) etc.

Alpha-1 receptor antagonists can cause *significant fluid retention and reduction in venous return* to the heart because of the peripheral vasodilation. Therefore, these drugs are generally administered *with caution in patients with congestive heart failure* and other fluid overloaded situations. Often a diuretic is also prescribed along with use of alpha-1 blockers to prevent complications from fluid retention. Common adverse reactions from alpha-1 blockers are *dizziness*, *fatigue*, *headache*, *peripheral edema*, *dose-related orthostatic hypotension*, *neuromuscular weakness*, *nasal congestion* etc.

Because of the effect of alpha-1 blockers on both prostate gland and vascular smooth muscle, *theoretically they are ideal choice for treatment of patients with both hypertension and benign prostatic hypertrophy*. However, when compared to other classes of antihypertensive agents like beta-blockers and calcium channel blockers, they are weak antihypertensive agents Hence, these drugs are *not used as first line agents for treatment of hypertension*.

Other beneficial effects of alpha-1 blockers come in the form of *reduction in total cholesterol and triglyceride levels along with increase in HDL*, *enhancing insulin sensitivity* and *improving activity of fibrinolytic system.* Therefore, these agents are useful for patients with diabetes, heart disease and high cholesterol. *Non steroidal Anti Inflammatory Drugs* (*NSAID*) *reduce the antihypertensive effect* of most of the alpha-1 blockers. Because of this reason, patients are instructed to avoid over the counter (OTC) drugs contain NSAIDs while taking alpha-1 blockers.

Centrally Acting Alpha-2 Agonist

As mentioned in the earlier part of this chapter, *activation of alpha-2 receptors result in the relaxation of smooth muscles*. Centrally acting alpha-2 agonist agents like **Clonidine** and **Methyldopa** are used in treatment of hypertension because of their *inhibitory effect in the cardio acceleration and vasoconstriction centers of the brain stem*. This action reduces flow of **Norepinephrine** in the periphery, leading to reduction in peripheral and renal vascular resistance, heart rate and blood pressure. This group of medications are used as *second-line agents for treatment of hypertension*. Common examples and their implications in clinical situations are described in the tables.

Drug	Onset of action	Half life	Metabolism	Elimination
Clonidine *Catapress®*	Oral 0.5-1 hr	12-16 hrs Up to 41 hrs (renal dysfunction)	Extensive hepatic	Urine
	Transdermal 2- 3 days	20 hrs		
Methyldopa *Aldomet®*	4-6 hrs	1.5 - 2 hrs Prolonged in renal disease	Intestinal and hepatic	Urine
Guanfacine *Tenex®*	2- 5 hrs	10-30 hrs	Hepatic	Urine
Guanabenz	60 min	6 hrs	Liver	Urine

Table 2.3. Pharmacokinetics of centrally acting Alpha 2 agonists

Clonidine activates alpha-2 receptors in the medulla of the brain and thereby *reducing sympathetic tone and increasing parasympathetic response*. This results in reduction of blood pressure and cause bradycardia. At the same time, Clonidine stimulates peripheral alpha-2 receptors causing vasodilation. **Clonidine** *does not cause significant orthostatic changes in blood pressure* because of its action on both central and peripheral receptors. Both Clonidine and Methyldopa reduce renal vascular resistance and thereby increases blood flow to the kidneys. This also helps in limiting **Renin Angiotensin Aldosterone system** (**RAAS**) activation.

Clinical Use of Centrally Acting Alpha-2 Agonists

Drug	Clinical Indication
Clonidine	Hypertension Hypertensive urgency* Nicotine and heroin withdrawal symptoms* Pain management (epidural injection)*
Methyldopa	Hypertension Hypertension in pregnancy
Guanfacine	Hypertension ADHD (in children)*
Guanabenz	Hypertension

* Off label use

Table 2.4. Clinical use of centrally acting Alpha 2 agonists

Adverse Effects of Centrally Acting Alpha 2 Agonists

Common adverse reactions of **Clonidine** are drowsiness, dry mouth, urinary retention, pruritic rashes, nightmares and insomnia. **Methyldopa** has been associated with development of **positive Coombs test** within 6 to 12 months after initiation of therapy. Positive Coombs test denotes possibility of IgG auto antibodies that are responsible for hemolytic anemia. In actuality, only a small percentage of people undergoing treatment with Methyldopa develop hemolytic anemia. Instruct the patients that while taking methyldopa, the urine left standing may turn dark red. This doesn't suggest having hematuria. These medications can *cause fluid retention and therefore should be used with caution* in patients with *congestive heart failure or severe renal dysfunction*.

Centrally acting alpha-2 agonists have *additive effect on central nervous system suppression* when used with agents like alcohol, antihistamines, phenothiazines, barbiturates and benzodiazepine. Centrally acting agents should be used with caution in patients with cerebrovascular disease and depression. It should also be used with caution in presence of severe coronary insufficiency, renal dysfunction and recent myocardial infarction.

One of the major clinical consideration for centrally acting alpha-2 agonists is that *sudden withdrawal of these agents can cause life-threatening rebound hypertension* produced from increased sympathetic nervous system activity. **Clonidine** and **Methyldopa** carries considerable risk of having this **rebound hypertension**. Therefore, discontinuation of these agents should be done gradually with tapering doses. It is believed that because of the relatively short half-life of Clonidine, inhibition of Norepinephrine release suddenly disappears after it's discontinuation. This leads to a sudden influx of sympathetic over activity causing rebound hypertension. *Re-introduction of Clonidine and start slow tapering dose is the ideal treatment*.

Nonselective Alpha Receptor Antagonist

Phentolamine (**OraVerse®**) is a non-selective alpha receptor antagonist commonly used in acute care settings because of its beneficial vasodilator effects. It *competitively blocks alpha receptors and thereby reduces circulating epinephrine and norepinephrine, leading to vasodilation*. Phentolamine is indicated for treatment of *extravasation with sympathomimetic drugs* like Dopamine, Dobutamine, Epinephrine, Norepinephrine and Vasopressin. Phentolamine is given through *local subcutaneous injection* in this situation. It reverses severe peripheral vasoconstriction induced by the vasoactive agents and thereby providing a window for "washout" of the drug from the local tissue that in turn prevents tissue necrosis. *Phentolamine should be given as early as possible* for optimal outcomes. In an off label basis, this drug is also used for treatment of pheochromocytoma and hypertensive crisis.

Points to remember!!!

- *Sympathetic nervous system helps with excitation and parasympathetic dealt with inhibition or down regulation of various functions.*
- Adrenergic agents *facilitate sympathetic nervous system activity*

by combining with sympathetic receptors such as **Alpha-1**, **Alpha-2**, **Beta-1**and **Beta-2** receptors.

- Alpha-1 adrenergic antagonists *selectively block Alpha-1 receptors in the vascular smooth muscle* and thereby reduce peripheral vascular resistance.
- Alpha-1 adrenergic antagonists *cause reduction in both arterial and venous vascular tone irrespective of the position of the patient* and may cause **orthostatic hypotension**.
- Alpha-1 receptor antagonists can cause *significant fluid retention and reduction in venous return* to the heart because of their peripheral vasodilation.
- Common adverse reactions from alpha-1 blockers are *dizziness, fatigue, headache, peripheral edema, dose-related orthostatic hypotension, neuromuscular weakness, nasal congestion* etc.
- Alpha-1 receptor antagonists are weak antihypertensive agents and hence *not used as first line agents for treatment of hypertension*.
- Beneficial effects of alpha-1 blockers comes in the form of *reduction in total cholesterol and triglyceride levels along with increase in HDL, enhancing insulin sensitivity* and *improving activity of fibrinolytic system.*
- *Non steroidal Anti Inflammatory Drugs* (*NSAID*) *reduce the antihypertensive effect* of most of the alpha-1 blockers
- Centrally acting alpha-2 agonist agents such as **Clonidine** and **Methyldopa** can cause inhibitory *effect in the cardio acceleration and vasoconstriction centers of the brain stem*.
- This action reduces flow of **Norepinephrine** in the periphery; leading to reduction in peripheral and renal vascular resistance, heart rate and blood pressure.
- Clonidine activates alpha-2 receptors in the medulla of the brain and thereby *reducing sympathetic tone and increasing parasympathetic response* and at the same time, Clonidine stimulates peripheral alpha-2 receptors causing vasodilation.
- Clonidine and Methyldopa reduce renal vascular resistance and

thereby increases blood flow to the kidneys and limit **Renin Angiotensin Aldosterone system** (**RAAS**) activation.

- Common adverse reactions of **Clonidine** are drowsiness, dry mouth, urinary retention, pruritic rashes, nightmares and insomnia.

- **Methyldopa** has been associated with development of **positive Coombs test** within 6 to 12 months after initiation of therapy.

- Alpha-2 agonist agents can *cause fluid retention and therefore should be used with caution* in patients with *congestive heart failure or severe renal dysfunction*

- Centrally acting alpha-2 agonists have *additive effect on central nervous system suppression* when used with agents like alcohol, antihistamines, phenothiazines

- *Sudden withdrawal of* alpha-2 agonists *can cause life-threatening rebound hypertension* produced from increased sympathetic nervous system activity.

- Therefore, discontinuation of these agents should be done gradually with tapering doses.

- *Reintroduction of Clonidine and start slow tapering dose is the ideal treatment for rebound hypertension from rapid drug withdrawal.*

- *Phentolamine competitively blocks alpha receptors and thereby reduce circulating epinephrine and norepinephrine; leading to vasodilation.*

- Phentolamine is indicated for treatment of *extravasation with sympathomimetic drugs* through *local subcutaneous injection.*

- In an off label basis, Phentolamine is also used for treatment of pheochromocytoma and hypertensive crisis.

3 Beta Receptor Blockers

Beta receptor blockers are one of the most important group of medications used in day-to-day cardiology practice. They are useful not only for cardiac disorders, but also for other diseases like glaucoma, migraine headache, hyperthyroidism, stage fright, alcohol withdrawal etc. Even though all these drugs are classified as 'beta-blockers', many of the newer generation agents have clinical properties that are not essentially beta receptor mediated. Some of them have properties which are not even explainable in terms of beta receptor activity!

Physiologically, *beta receptors are stimulated by catecholamines as a result of sympathetic nervous system activity*. There are mainly two groups of beta receptors known as **beta-1** and **beta-2 receptors**. The concentration of these receptors in different organs can vary depending on the clinical situation. In general, some organs are primarily stimulated by beta-1 receptors and others by beta-2 receptors. *At lower concentration*, *many of the beta-blockers can selectively act on either beta-1 or beta-2 receptors*. Some of these agents have a small amount of *sympathetic nervous system stimulation along with beta blockade activity*. This property is

> Agents with **intrinsic sympathomimetic activity** (**ISA**) exerts low level of beta receptor stimulation along with their beta receptor blockade depending on the available amount of the drug as well as the hormones (e.g. Norepinephrine) against which the drug is working. For example, Acebutolol and Pindolol; at rest they act as beta stimulants. However during activity where intrinsic (natural) beta stimulation is high, they act as beta blockers.
>
> One clinical scenario for beneficial use of this function is a patient who has significant resting bradycardia requiring beta blocker therapy. Drugs with ISA may prevent resting bradycardia through stimulation rather than inhibition of beta receptors; however, suppress beta receptors during exercise to reduce heart rate and myocardial oxygen demand.

Receptor	Organs
Beta-1*	Heart Intestine Kidney(Renin producing tissue) Adipose tissue Brain Eyes (aqueous humor producing cells)
Beta-2*	Bronchial and vascular smooth muscle Gastro Intestinal tract Uterus Insulin secreting cells of pancreas Liver

*It is important to note that none of the organs exclusively contain either beta-1 or beta-2 receptors.

Table 3.1 Beta receptors in various organs

known as **intrinsic sympathomimetic activity** (**ISA**) and is seen in **Acebutolol** and **Pindolol**. This knowledge about receptor selectivity and other characteristics are put to use in identifying specific beta-blocker agents for specific clinical scenarios.

Action of Beta Receptors

In order to communicate commands from central or autonomic nervous system to the target cells, body has a number of electrical and chemical pathways connecting the origin of the impulse to the responding tissue. In simple terms, *receptors act as part of the gatekeeper and message decoding system* in many of the cell membranes. They help in identifying chemical messages produced by various nervous system terminals. These gatekeepers, when stimulated by appropriate chemicals initiate a chain of actions within the cell by interacting with other biochemical molecules. This process results in electrochemical changes at the cellular level as in the case of opening specific

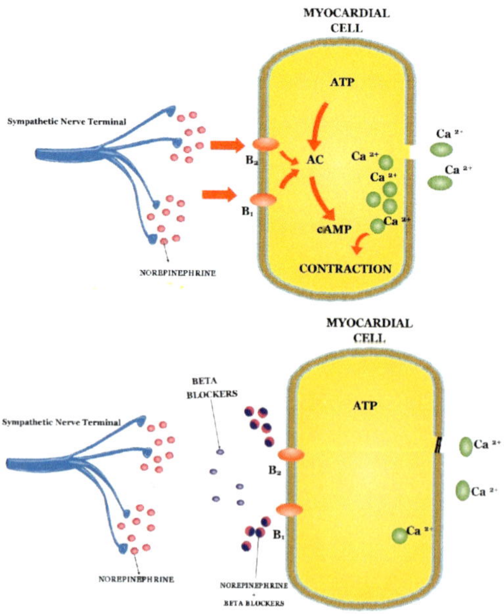

Fig 3.1 Beta receptors and the heart

pathways for electrolyte ions. The entire process can be easily explained through the following example.

In cardiac cells, beta receptors situated on the cell membrane are stimulated by **Norepinephrine**, which is a chemical neurotransmitter from sympathetic nervous system terminal. The stimulation of beta receptor by Norepinephrine initiates activation of **Adenyl Cyclase**, which is a regulatory protein within the cell. The stimulation of Adenyl Cyclase (AC) activates production of **cyclic Adenosine Monophosphate** (**cAMP**) and that in turn stimulate *opening of calcium channels* to let more calcium ions in to the cell. This influx of calcium ions cause increase in contractility of the cardiac cells, which is the net effect of beta stimulation in the myocardial tissue.

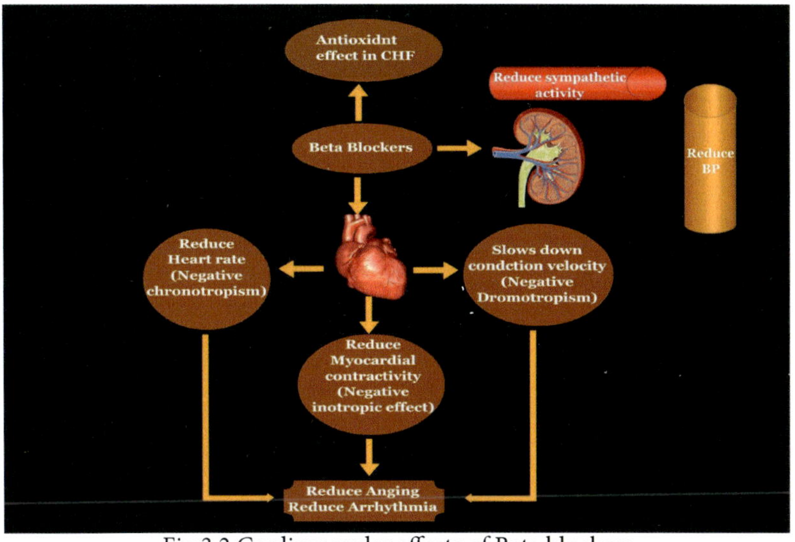

Fig 3.2 Cardiovascular effects of Beta blockers

Beta-blocker medications *mimic the chemical structure of catecholamines and thereby competitively attached to the receptors* and block the initiation of chemical messenger system. Hence they terminate the effect of sympathetic nervous system on the target organ. As these agents are competitive inhibitors, *adequate concentration of the drug at the receptor site is essential for the desired effect*.

Cardiac tissues contain predominantly **beta-1 receptors** (*70:30 ratios between the number of beta-1 and beta-2 receptors*). The effect of beta-1 receptor blockade is described as follows.

Drug	Onset of action	Half life	Metabolism	Elimination
Acebutolol *Sectral®*	1 to 2 hours	3 to 4 hours	Extensive first pass	Renal
Metoprolol *Toprol ®*	1.5 to 4 hours (oral) 20 min (IV)	3 to 8 hours	Significant first pass	Hepatic
Propranolol *Inderal®*	1 to 2 hours	3 to 6 hours	Extensive first pass	Hepatic
Timolol	15 to 45 min	2 to 2.5 hours	Extensive first pass	Hepatic
Esmolol *Brevibloc®*	2 to 10 min (IV)	9 min	By red blood cell esterase	Renal
Atenolol *Tenormin ®*	2 to 4 hours	6 to 7 hours 15 to 35 hours (renal impairment)	Limited hepatic	Renal
Carvedilol *Coreg®*	1 to 2 hours	7-10 hours	Extensive hepatic	Hepatic
Labetalol *Trandate®*	20 to 120 min (oral) 2 to 5 min (IV)	6 to 8 hours	Extensive first pass	Hepatic and renal
Sotalol *Betapace®*	1 to 2 hours (oral) 5 to 10 min (IV)	12 hours up to 48 hours (in severe renal impairment)	No hepatic metabolism	Renal
Bisoprolol *Zebeta®*	1 to 2 hours	9-12 hours	Significant first pass	Renal and hepatic
Nadolol *Corgard ®*	2 to 4 hours	10 to 24 hours up to 45 hours (in severe renal impairment)	Not metabolized	Renal

Table 3.2 Pharmacokinetics of Beta blockers

1. Reduce heart rate (negative **Chronotropic effect**), decrease myocardial contractility (negative **Inotropic effect**), slows down conduction velocity (negative **Dromotropic effect**). These effects together help to reduce incidence of angina and arrhythmias (especially those induced by increased catecholamine levels and presence of re-entry circuits like paroxysmal supraventricular tachycardia [PSVT]).

2. They interfere with sympathetic vasoconstrictor activity in the peripheral vessels and reduce Renin release from Juxtaglomerular cells of the kidney. These actions effectively cause *reduction in blood pressure*.

3. Some of the newer generation beta-blockers like **Carvedilol** have potent antioxidant effects that prevent catecholamine toxicity of the myocardial tissue especially in the event of congestive heart failure (CHF).

Drug	Beta Selectivity	Uses
Propranolol (Inderal)	Non-selective beta-blocker	Hypertension Migraine prophylaxis Essential tremor Hypertrophic sub aortic stenosis Pheochromocytoma Tachyarrhythmia Thyroid storm and thyrotoxicosis (off label)
Timolol	Nonselective beta-blocker	Anti-Glaucoma (topical) Hypertension Prevention of MI Migraine prophylaxis
Nadolol (Corgard)	Non-selective beta-blocker	Angina pectoris Hypertension Variceal hemorrhage prophylaxis (off label)
Sotalol (Betapace)	Nonselective beta-blocker and class III antiarrhythmic agent	Atrial fibrillation or flutter Ventricular tachycardia
Atenolol (Tenormin)	Beta-1 selective	Hypertension Angina pectoris Post myocardial infarction Thyrotoxicosis (off label)
Metoprolol (Lopressor, Toprol-XL)	Beta -1 selective	Angina pectoris Atrial fibrillation or flutter Supra ventricular tachycardia Hypertension Heart failure (Toprol XL) Thyrotoxicosis (off label)
Bisoprolol (Zebeta)	Beta-1 selective	Hypertension Heart failure (off label)
Esmolol (Brevibloc) (available only as injection or infusion)	Beta-1 selective	Supraventricular tachycardia Atrial fibrillation or flutter Intra or post operative tachycardia and hypertension
Acebutolol (Sectral)	Beta-1 selective with intrinsic sympathomimetic activity (ISA)	Hypertension Angina pectoris Ventricular arrhythmias Chronic stable angina (off label)
Nebivolol (Bystolic)	Beta -1 selective with Nitric oxide mediated vasodilator property	Hypertension Heart failure (off label)
Carvedilol (Coreg)	Non selective beta blocking with alpha blocking activity	Hypertension Heart failure LV dysfunction following MI Angina pectoris (off label)
Labetalol (Trandate)	Non selective beta blocker with alpha blocker property	Hypertension Hypertensive urgency Arterial hypertension in acute ischemic stroke(off label)

Table 3.4.Clinical application of Beta blockers

Apart from beta -1 and beta-2 selectivity of earlier generation beta-blockers, the newer generation agents such as **Carvedilol** and **Labetalol** have *both alpha and beta blockade effect*. Especially Carvedilol that is approved for treatment of congestive heart failure, reduces blood pressure by initiating peripheral vasodilation without significant reduction in cardiac output. However, these agents *can cause orthostatic hypotension*. **Nebivolol** is the *most beta-1 selective* and newest beta-blocker with a property of *Nitric oxide mediated vasodilation*, which is different from all of the other beta-blockers.

Common clinical applications of betablockers are described in the table 3.4.

Major Side Effects of Beta-Blockers

The most important and common adverse reactions from beta blockers are *hypotension and bradycardia*. These symptoms are produced as a direct effect of beta blocking activity in the cardiac system. Therefore, beta-blockers are *used with caution* in patients with underlying low blood pressure, bradycardia, various degree of heart blocks other than first degree heart block unless there is a pacemaker, sick sinus syndrome etc.

Common Side Effects of Beta Blockers

- Fatigue
- Hypotension
- Bradycardia
- Broncho constriction
- Masking of hypoglycemia
- Slows recovery from hypoglycemia
- Increase triglycerides and reduce HDL*
- Orthostatic hypotension*

* Mainly with Carvedilol and Labetalol

Box 3.1 Common side effects of Beta blockers

Even though widely used in day-to-day clinical practice, beta-blockers may produce serious side effects not only in cardiovascular system but also in other organs. These side effects are the common reasons for non-compliance with beta blockers. Many of the events are associated with normal beta blocking pharmacologic action. Some of them can be avoided by using selective beta receptor agents. However, it is interesting to note that in *higher doses, these medications lose their receptor selectivity* and

Contraindications for Beta-blocker Therapy	
Do not use	☒ Severe bradycardia ☒ Severe conduction system disease (Sick sinus syndrome or high-grade AV block) ☒ Severe bronchospasm or airway disease ☒ Severe peripheral vascular disease ☒ Cardiogenic shock ☒ Cocaine induced tachycardia* (*Cause unopposed alpha stimulation)
Use with caution	☒ Hypotension ☒ Mild asthma or severe COPD ☒ Reynaud's phenomena ☒ Vasospastic angina ☒ Insulin-dependent diabetes mellitus with frequent hypoglycemia ☒ Pregnancy ☒ Sexual dysfunction ☒ Excessive fatigue and weakness

Box 3.2 Contraindications for Beta blocker therapy

can affect beta receptors indiscriminately.

For example, action of beta-blockers in the lungs can interfere with normal bronchodilator activity. This may produce bronco-constriction, which is detrimental for patients with reactive airway disease like asthma or advanced chronic obstructive pulmonary disease (COPD). Since beta-2 receptors are predominantly seen in the lungs, *use of a cardio selective beta -1 antagonist agent* can abate these potential side-effects.

Similarly, *beta-blocker effect on the insulin secreting cells of the pancreas* can reduce insulin production and thereby *hinder the recovery from hypoglycemia* in patients with type-II diabetes. Beta-blockers can also *mask the symptoms of hypoglycemia* except diaphoresis. This is due to the fact that *most of the hypoglycemic symptoms are driven by sympathetic nervous system stimulation*, which is blocked by the use of beta blockers. Therefore, beta blockers should be used with caution in patients with type-II Diabetes Mellitus.

Fatigue, depression, weakness, insomnia and vivid dreams are seen as part of central nervous system side effects. These symptoms are *significant in beta-blockers with high lipid solubility* like Carvedilol, Propranolol, Timolol, Nebivolol and Metoprolol. This phenomenon is *due to the higher concentration of these drugs in the brain*, as lipid soluble drugs can easily pass blood brain barrier compared to the water-soluble agents like Atenolol and Sotalol. The side effect of fatigue is believed to be a consequence of decreased cardiac output as part of beta-blocker effect.

Non-selective beta-blockers can increase triglyceride levels and reduce HDL and therefore used with caution in patients with underlying disorders of lipid metabolism. *Sudden withdrawal of beta-blockers can precipitate angina pectoris* or even myocardial infarction in patients with significant coronary disease. This is because of the sudden beta receptor stimulation that was previously cordoned by beta-blockers. Patients with **pheochromocytoma** *should be treated with caution* using beta-blockers *because of the unopposed Alpha adrenergic stimulation*, which is part of the disease process. This may cause **hypertensive crisis**. Treatment options of beta blocker toxicity are described in the box.

Treatment of Beta Blocker Toxicity

- Intravenous Atropine or temporary pacemaker (for severe bradycardia)
- IV dextrose and IV glucagon (for symptomatic hypoglycemia)
- Infusion of Isoproterenol (Isuprel®)
- High dose Dobutamine infusion (15 mcg/kg/min)
- IV Calcium chloride(1 gm over 10 min) or Calcium gluconate
- High dose insulin and glucose
- Magnesium (for ventricular arrhythmias especially with Sotalol)

Box 3.3 Treatment of Beta blocker toxicity

Points to remember!!!

- *Beta receptors are stimulated by catecholamines as a result of sympathetic nervous system activity.*
- In general, some organs are primarily stimulated by beta-1 receptors and others by beta-2 receptors.
- *At lower concentration, many of the beta-blockers can selectively act on either beta-1 or beta-2 receptors.*

- Agents like **Acebutolol** and **Pindolol** have a small amount of *sympathetic nervous system stimulation along with beta blockade activity and* is known as **intrinsic sympathomimetic activity(ISA)**

- **Beta-blocker medications** *mimic the chemical structure of catecholamines and thereby competitively attach to the receptors* and block the initiation of chemical messenger system.

- Cardiac tissue contain predominantly **beta-1 receptors**

- Beta-1 receptor blockade on cardiac cells cause reduction in heart rate (negative **chronotropic effect**), decrease in myocardial contractility (negative **inotropic effect**) and slows down conduction velocity (negative **dromotropic effect**).

- Beta-1 receptor blockers interfere with sympathetic vasoconstrictor activity in the peripheral vessels and also reduce Renin release from Juxtaglomerular cells of the kidney and effectively cause *reduction in blood pressure*.

- Beta blockers like Carvedilol has potent antioxidant effects that prevent catecholamine toxicity of the myocardial tissue especially in the event of congestive heart failure

- **Carvedilol** and **Labetalol** have *both alpha and beta blockade effect*.

- **Nebivolol** is the *most beta-1 selective* and newest beta-blocker with a property of *Nitric oxide mediated vasodilation*,

- The most important and common adverse reactions from beta blockers are *hypotension and bradycardia*.

- In *higher doses, beta blockers lose their receptor selectivity* and can affect beta receptors indiscriminately.

- Since beta-2 receptors are predominantly seen in the lungs, *use of a cardio selective beta -1 antagonist agent is preferred in advanced lung disease like COPD*

- *Beta blocker effect on the insulin secreting cells of the pancreas* can reduce insulin production and thereby *hinder the recovery from hypoglycemia* in patients with type-II diabetes

- Beta-blockers can also *mask the symptoms of hypoglycemia* except diaphoresis.
- Fatigue, depression, weakness, insomnia and vivid dreams are seen as side effects and are believed to be *significant in beta-blockers with high lipid solubility* such as Carvedilol, Propranolol, Timolol, Nebivolol and Metoprolol.
- *Non-selective beta-blockers can increase triglyceride levels and reduce HDL*
- *Sudden withdrawal of beta-blockers can precipitate angina pectoris*
- Patients with **pheochromocytoma** *should be treated with caution* using beta-blockers *because of the unopposed Alpha adrenergic stimulat*ion, which is part of the disease process and may cause **hypertensive crisis**.

4 Calcium Channel Blockers

Calcium channel blockers (CCB) are commonly used for treatment of hypertension, vasospasm, and arrhythmias. These agents achieve their pharmacologic action through *blockade of entry channels for calcium into the intracellular environment*. Calcium ions are the essential elements in maintaining contractility of all muscle groups, especially the smooth muscles. *The amount of intracellular calcium ions directly relates to the strength of muscle contraction*. There are two different types of calcium channels exist in the plasma membrane, **L type** and **T type**. **L Type** channels are capable of responding to the sympathetic nervous system stimulation. **T type** channels have a role in controlling the depolarization of SA node, AV node and other conduction system tissues.

The calcium channel blocking actions of all the available Calcium channel blockers are through both 'voltage gated' and 'receptor operated' channels. Interestingly, since the L type channels are stimulated by sympathetic stimulation, Beta blockers can also affect these receptor sites and impart some calcium channel blocking effect.

All of the Calcium channel blockers available today have effect on L types channels and a selective group has effect on the T type channel. This channel specificity determines clinical effect of various drugs in this class. Calcium channel blockers are mainly classified based on the receptor sites where they impart inward calcium regulation.

Classification of Calcium Channel Blockers

In general, Calcium channel blockers are classified in to two types depending on the type of calcium channels they interact. They are Type I calcium channel blockers (Non-dihydropyridines) and Type II calcium channel blocker (Dihydropyridines). The channel selectivity and examples of these agents are shown in the box.

Type	Channel Selectivity	Example
Non-dihydropyridines	L -type channel blockers along with some T- Type channel blocking property	Verapamil Diltiazem
Dihydropyridines	selective L type channel blockers	Amlodipine Felodipine Nifedipine Nicardipine Nimodipine Nisoldipine

Box 4.1.Types of Calcium channel blockers

Non-dihydropyridines: Because of the *predominant effect in the cardiac conduction system*, non-dihydropyridine (non-DHP) calcium channel blockers are mainly *used for management of arrhythmias* (*negative chronotropic effect*). This group of drugs not only block the calcium channels, but also slows down the recovery of calcium channels in the SA and AV nodal tissue. This process results in *reduced automaticity and conductivity within the nodes*. This explains the beneficial effect of Non-dihydropyridine agents in management of tachycardia.

Dihydropyridine (DHP) calcium channel blockers: They impart *negative ionotropic effect* and thereby reduce contractility of myocardium through regulation of calcium ions into the myocardial cells. This group of drugs also cause relaxation of peripheral arterial smooth muscles, leading to *afterload reduction without affecting cardiac preload* (because they do not dilate veins). They are commonly used for management of hypertension, angina pectoris etc.

Dihydropyridine (DHP) group of Calcium channel blockers (e.g. Amlodipine, Nifedipine) are potent vasodilators with less electrophysiologic and cardio depressive functions compared to Verapamil and Diltiazem (non-dihydropyridine).

Pharmacokinetics

All Calcium channel blockers are *well absorbed through oral administration* and have major hepatic metabolism through **CYP3A4 isoenzymes**. Presence of *food in the gut does not affect* the absorption or bioavailability however, food items like **grapefruit** juice that are *potential inhibitors of CYP3A4 isoenzymes system* may affect the availability of the free drug. High-fat and high carbohydrate meal can also affect active drug availability of some Calcium channel blockers. Most of the agents are metabolized through liver and excreted through urine and feces. Majority of calcium channel blockers except Amlodipine and extended-release (ER or XL) preparations have shorter half-life of around 2 to 8 hours. *Amlodipine has a half-life of 30 to 50 hours*.

Drug	Onset	Half Life	Metabolism	Elimination
Verapamil *Calan®* *Isoptin®*	1 to 2 hours (oral) 1 to 5 min (IV)	5 to 12 hours 14 to 16 hours (severe hepatic dysfunction)	Extensive first pass	Hepatic and renal
Diltiazem *Cardizem®* *Cartia-XT®*	30 to 60 min (oral) 3 min (IV)	3 to 4 hours (immediate release) 5to 10 hours (extended-release)	Extensive first pass	Hepatic
Amlodipine *Norvasc®*	1 to 2 hours	30 to 50 hours	Hepatic	Hepatic
Felodipine *Plendil®*	2 to 5 hours	11 to 16 hours	Extensive first pass	Hepatic and renal
Nicardipine *Cardene®*	0.5 to 2 hrs	2 to 4 hours	Extensive first pass	Hepatic and renal
Nifedipine *Adalat®* *Procardia®*	20 min	2 to 5 hours	Hepatic	Hepatic
Nimodipine *Nimotop®*	Within 1 hour	1 to 2 hours	Extensive hepatic	Hepatic
Isradipine *Dynacirc CR®*	2 to 3 hours	8 hours	Extensive first pass	Hepatic and renal

Table 4.1. Pharmacokinetics of Calcium channel blockers

Non-dihydropyridine calcium channel blockers are *contraindicated after significant myocardial infarction especially in patients with depressed Left Ventricular function*. This is because of the **negative ionotropic effect** in the heart that can further worsen associated congestive heart failure. However, type II (Dihydropyridine) Calcium channel blockers like Amlodipine can be useful because of the strong peripheral vasodilator property than the depressing effect on the heart to achieve desired outcomes.

Drug	Property	Clinical use
Verapamil	Non DHP	Angina pectoris Chronic Atrial fibrillation (for rate control) PSVT prophylaxis Hypertension Supra Ventricular Tachycardia (SVT)
Diltiazem	Non DHP	Angina pectoris Hypertension Atrial Fibrillation Atrial flutter Paroxysmal Supra Ventricular Tachycardia(PSVT)
Amlodipine	DHP	Hypertension Angina Pectoris
Felodipine	DHP	Hypertension
Nimodipine	DHP	Vasospasm following Subarachnoid hemorrhage (SAH)
Nicardipine	DHP	Hypertension Hypertensive emergency (IV) Angina pectoris Arterial hypertension in acute ischemic stroke
Nifedipine	DHP	Chronic stable angina Vasospastic angina Hypertension Pulmonary hypertension** Raynaud's phenomena**
Isradipine	DHP	Hypertension

** Off label use

Table 4.2.Clinical use of Calcium channel blockers

Since Calcium channel blockers can cause smooth muscle relaxation, they should be *used with caution in patients with gastro-esophageal reflux disease* (GERD).In these patients, Calcium channel blockers can relax esophageal sphincter and thereby worsen the symptoms of GERD.

Adverse Effects and Interactions

Major side effects of Calcium channel blockers *include headache*, *dizziness*, *hypotension*, *syncope*, *flushing* and *peripheral edema*. All of these effects can be traced back to the vasodilator property of Calcium channel blockers. Short-acting forms of Calcium channel blockers are generally avoided except for acute rhythm control in clinical settings because of the higher side-effect profile. Some of these agents, especially **Verapamil** may cause gastro intestinal (GI) side effects like constipation, nausea and vomiting. Caution should be used while administering Calcium channel blockers along with other antihypertensive medications because the *additive effect can produce profound hypotension*.

Contraindication for CCB

- WPW syndrome
- Severe left ventricular dysfunction
- Digitalis toxicity
- Severe constipation (Verapamil)
- Severe aortic stenosis
- Severe sinus node dysfunction and conduction system disease

Box 4.2. Contraindications for Calcium blockers

Non-dihydropyridine (Non DHP) calcium channel blockers, especially **Verapamil** can cause serious rhythm disturbances like *second or third degree heart block, ventricular conduction defects and prolonged PR interval*. As mentioned earlier, because of the cardio depressive nature (negative ionotropic effect), Non DHP agents should be used with caution in patients with severe left ventricular dysfunction (low ejection fraction). Non DHP calcium channel blockers *should not be used for rate control in patients with atrial fibrillation* associated with the **Wolf Parkinson white** (**WPW**) **syndrome** as it can cause lethal tachyarrhythmia.

Calcium Channel Blocker Toxicity Treatment

- Atropine (for symptomatic bradycardia)
- Intravenous Calcium
- Glucagon (increases intracellular cAMP levels and improves heart rate)
- Vasopressors (direct-acting agent with positive inotropic, positive chronotropic, and vasoconstrictive effects. E.g. Norepinephrine or Levophed)
- High-dose insulin and glucose (positive inotropic effect)

Box 4.3.Management of Calcium channel blocker toxicity

Verapamil when used with **Digoxin** can increase Digoxin level and therefore need close monitoring. Since these medications are metabolized through **CYP3A4 enzyme** system, they can *potentially increase the blood level* of other drugs like **Statins**, **Theophylline**, **Carbamazepine** etc.

Clinical Usage

Chronic Stable Angina

Peripheral vasodilatation along with negative chronotropic effects of calcium channel blockers help in *reducing oxygen demand of myocardial tissue*. They also *cause coronary vasodilation* leading to better coronary perfusion. *Extended-Release preparations of calcium channel blockers* except Amlodipine are *used to avoid* **reflex tachycardia**, which may make anginal symptoms worse. Because of the long half life of Amlodipine, reflex tachycardia incidents are at a minimum. Verapamil (non-DHP) is not commonly used in patients with associated LV dysfunction because of reduction in myocardial contractility secondary to its strong negative ionotropic effect. However, *Diltiazem is of the same class but having less negative ionotropic effect can be used in these patients* who need heart rate control. Calcium channel blockers, especially the short-acting formulations are not recommended for patients with known coronary artery disease. This is because they can worsen symptoms by increasing myocardial oxygen demand through sympathetic stimulation and reflux tachycardia, unless used with a beta-blocker.

Hypertension

Calcium channel blockers, especially Dihydropyridines are cornerstone in hypertension treatment. These agents are used in conjunction with Beta-blockers, ACE inhibitors or Diuretics. They have better clinical effect in **African-American population** than many of the other agents in controlling hypertension. They lower blood pressure mainly by *relaxing arterial smooth muscle and thereby reducing peripheral vascular resistance*. Long acting preparations provide stable blood pressure control around-the-clock along with fewer side effects induced by sympathetic stimulation like reflux tachycardia. Hence, they have a better compliance and tolerability among patients. Calcium channel blockers are more appropriate in patients with contraindication for use of beta-blockers like severe airway disease for treatment of hypertension.

Atrial Arrhythmias

Non-Dihydropyridine calcium channel blockers (Verapamil and Diltiazem) are indicated for treatment of supraventricular tachycardia (SVT) because of the predominant effect in the conduction system. They *lower automaticity and conductivity of nodal tissue* and thereby control heart rate in tachyarrhythmias. As mentioned earlier, Verapamil has significant negative ionotropic effect compared to Diltiazem and therefore is not suitable for patients with underlying left ventricular dysfunction. In acute care setting, short-acting intravenous preparations of these agents are used for rate control in patients with paroxysmal supraventricular tachycardia or atrial fibrillation/flutter with rapid ventricular response. They do not impart any effect on conversion of atrial fibrillation to sinus rhythm. Since it only affects the nodal tissue, *Verapamil should not be used for rate control in patients with tachycardia involving accessory pathways* (eg. atrial fibrillation with WPW syndrome) . In these patients, slowing of AV nodal conduction by Verapamil may accelerate impulse propagation through accessory pathway resulting in lethal ventricular arrhythmias.

Ischemic Heart Disease

Because of the vasodilator property and reduction in contractility, Calcium channel blockers can *prevent exercise induced coronary vasoconstriction* and *reduce myocardial oxygen demand* along with *heart rate*. In **vasospastic angina** (**Prinzmetal's angina**), these agents are of excellent use because of the vasodilator effect that helps in preventing anginal attacks. However, in patients with known coronary artery disease, short-acting calcium channel blockers can produce reflux tachycardia and worsen symptoms. They are not used for routine prophylactic treatment for patients with myocardial infarction unless beta-blockers are contraindicated and have preserved left ventricular function.

Congestive Heart Failure

As mentioned earlier, heart failure patients with left ventricular dysfunction may have negative response from Calcium channel blockers because of the negative ionotropic effect. However, in patients with **left ventricular diastolic dysfunction** where *lack of sufficient ventricular relaxation is the underlying pathology*, Calcium channel blockers may provide beneficial effect *by augmenting ventricular relaxation and compliance along with heart rate control*. This action of Calcium Channel blockers help in improving ventricular filling. Because of the lack of sufficient evidence, *calcium channel blockers are not generally considered as first-line therapy for heart failure patients* irrespective of their ventricular function.

Other Disorders

Because of the effect of calcium blockers on smooth muscle relaxation, *Diltiazem has been used for patients with mild esophageal spasm* as an off label use. Diltiazem should be used with caution in patients with significant gastro-esophageal reflux disease (GERD) as it can worsen the symptoms. Because of the high affinity to the cerebral vessels, Nimodipine is used for treatment of cerebral vasospasm in patients with subarachnoid hemorrhage. Sustained release Verapamil is used for migraine headache prophylaxis as an off label use. Similarly, long acting Nifedipine is used for treatment of arterial spasm involving Raynaud's phenomena.

Points to remember!!!

- Calcium channel blockers achieve their pharmacologic action through *blockade of entry channels for calcium into the intracellular environment*.
- *The amount of intracellular calcium ions directly relates to the strength of muscle contraction*.
- **L Type** channels are capable of responding to the sympathetic nervous system response whereas **T type** channels have a role in controlling the depolarization of SA node, AV node and other conduction system tissues.
- All of the Calcium channel blockers available today have effect on L types channels and a selective group has effect on the T type channel.
- Calcium channel blockers are classified in to two typed depending on the type of calcium channels they interact and are Type I calcium channel blockers (Non-dihydropyridines) and Type II calcium channel blocker (Dihydropyridines).
- Non-dihydropyridine (non-DHP) calcium channel blockers are mainly *used for management of arrhythmias.*
- **Dihydropyridine (DHP) calcium channel blockers** impart *negative ionotropic effect* and thereby reduce contractility of myocardium
- This group of drugs also cause relaxation of peripheral arterial smooth muscles, leading to *afterload reduction without*

affecting cardiac preload

- All Calcium channel blockers are *well absorbed through oral administration* and have major hepatic metabolism through CYP3A4 **isoenzymes**.
- Food items like **grapefruit juice** which are *potential inhibitors of CYP3A4 isoenzymes system* may affect the availability of free drug.
- Majority of calcium channel blockers except Amlodipine have shorter half-life of around 2 to 8 hours. *Amlodipine has a half-life of 30 to 50 hours*.
- Non-dihydropyridine calcium channel blockers are *contraindicated after significant myocardial infarction especially in patients with depressed Left Ventricular function*
- Major side effects of Calcium channel blockers include *headache*, *dizziness*, *hypotension*, *syncope*, *flushing* and *peripheral edema*.
- **Verapamil** and Diltiazem can cause serious rhythm disturbances like *second or third degree heart block, ventricular conduction defects and prolonged PR interval*.
- Non DHP calcium channel blockers *should not be used for treatment of the rate control in patients with atrial fibrillation associated with* the **Wolf Parkinson white** (**WPW**) **syndrome**
- **Verapamil** when used with **Digoxin** can increase Digoxin level
- Peripheral vasodilatation along with negative chronotropic effects of calcium channel blockers helps in *reducing oxygen demand of myocardial tissue*.
- *Extended-Release preparations of calcium channel blockers* except Amlodipine are *used to avoid* **reflex tachycardia**,
- Non-Dihydropyridine calcium channel blockers (Verapamil and Diltiazem) are indicated for treatment of supraventricular tachycardia
- Calcium channel blockers can *prevent exercise induced coronary vasoconstriction* and *reduce myocardial oxygen demand*

- **In left ventricular diastolic dysfunction**, Calcium channel blockers may provide beneficial effect *by augmenting ventricular relaxation and compliance along with heart rate control* .

- *Calcium channel blockers are not generally considered as first-line therapy for heart failure patients*

- Because of the effect of calcium blockers on smooth muscle relaxation, *Diltiazem has been used for patients with mild esophageal spasm*

5 Renin- Angiotensin- Aldosterone system inhibitors

Renin- Angiotensin- Aldosterone System (RAAS) is one of the major chemical axis that has a *predominant role in maintaining peripheral vascular resistance and systemic blood pressure*. **Renin** is an enzyme secreted from **Juxtaglomerular cells** located in the **afferent arterioles** of the kidney. Production of Renin is *stimulated by* factors like *decreasing renal blood flow*, *hypotension*, *reduction in intravascular volume*, *sodium depletion* and *beta adrenergic stimulation*. You may see that all these stimulating events cause disturbance in stability of the vascular system and therefore Renin acts as a protective mechanism to reverse potential harmful effect from similar events. Formation of Renin initiates a cascade of processes that have widespread effect on various organ systems. Renin acts on **Angiotensinogen** and convert into **Angiotensin I**. This molecule itself is an inactive agent and is further converted into active **Angiotensin II**. This Angiotensin II has influence on multiple body systems including peripheral vasculature, renal tubules, adrenal gland, posterior pituitary etc. The effect of Angiotensin II is described in the table.

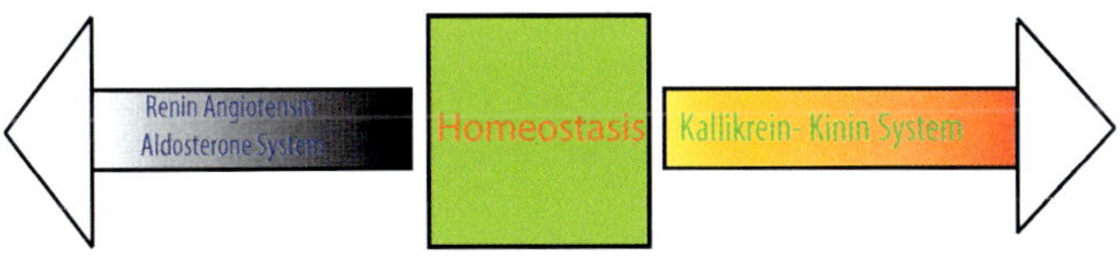

Fig 5.1 RAAS counterbalance system

Normal human physiology, effects of RAAS is counterbalanced by the **Kallikrein- Kinin system** to *prevent overstimulation from either of these entities*. This balance maintain normal blood pressure. Similar to **Angiotensin converting enzyme** (**ACE**) in RAAS system, activation of Kallikrein- Kinin system produce **Bradykinin**. The primary effect of Bradykinin in the circulatory system is that of *vasodilatation* and *excretion of sodium* (Natriuresis). Bradykinin, by nature is *an inflammatory mediator*

Organ	Effect of Angiotensin II	Effect of ACEI/ ARB
Peripheral arteries	Vasoconstriction (40 times stronger than norepinephrine) Increased peripheral vascular resistance and after load	vasodilation
Kidney	Enhance sodium reabsorption in proximal tubule	Enhance sodium excretion
Adrenal gland	Stimulate Aldosterone release from adrenal cortex Causing sodium and water retention and potassium excretion. Stimulate adrenal medulla to produce catecholamines.	Reduction in Aldosterone secretion causing sodium and water excretion and potassium retention.
Sympathetic nervous system	Stimulate sympathetic response	Reduce sympathetic stimulation
Pituitary gland	Enhance anti-diuretic hormone (ADH) secretion	Enhance free water loss
Smooth muscle	Enhance cell proliferation (Cause hypertrophy and remodeling)	Reduce remodeling (including myocardium)

Table 5.1.Effect of Angiotensin II and its antagonists in various organs

Drug	Onset	Half Life	Metabolism	Elimination
Captopril *Capoten®*	1-1.5 Hrs	1.9 hrs 20-40 hrs in anuria	Liver	Urine
Benazepril *Lotensin®*	1-2 hrs	10-11 hrs	Hepatic	Urine
Enalapril *Vasotec ®*	< 1hr	2 hrs	Hepatic	Urine
Quinapril *Accupril®*	1 hr	3 hrs	Liver	Urine
Fosinopril *Monopril®*	1 hr	12 hrs	Liver	Urine
Moexipril *Univasc ®*	1-2 hrs	2-9 hrs	Liver	Feces
Lisinopril *Prinivil ®*	1 hr	11-12 hr	Not metabolized	Urine
Perindopril *Aceon ®*	1-2 hr	3-10 hrs	Hepatic	Urine
Ramipril *Altace ®*	1-2 hrs	13-17 hrs	Hepatic	Urine
Trandalopril *Mavik®*	1-2 hr	22.5 hr	Hepatic	Urine

Table 5.2 Pharmacokinetics of ACEI

Drug	Onset	Half Life	Metabolism	Elimination
Angiotensin Receptor Blockers				
Losartan *Cozaar®*	6 hr	6-9 hr	Hepatic	Feces and Urine
Valsartan *Diovan®*	<2 hrs	<6 hr	Hepatic	Feces
Telmisartan *Micardis®*	1-2 hr	24 hr	Hepatic	Feces
Olmesartan Benicar®	1-2 hr	13 hr	No metabolism	Feces and Urine
Irbesartan *Avapro®*	1-2 hr	11-15 hr	Hepatic	Feces and Urine
Candesartan *Atacand®*	2-3 hr	5-9 hr	Liver	Feces and urine
Eprosartan *Teveten®*	1-2 hr	5-9 hr	Liver	Feces
Azilsartan *Edarbi®*	1.5-3 hr	11 hr	Hepatic	Feces and Urine
Direct Renin Inhibitor				
Aliskerin *Tekturna®*	1-3 hr	16-32 hr	Liver	Urine and feces

Table 5.3 Pharmacokinetics of ARB and Direct renin inhibitors

and works with **prostaglandin** *to produce pain* and *extra vascular smooth muscle contraction*. **Angiotensin converting enzyme** *facilitates the degradation of Bradykinin* and keep these action at minimal levels. Inhibition of Angiotensin converting enzyme helps to promote Bradykinin activity.

Bradykinin facilitates excretion of sodium and water through preventing stimulation of Aldosterone production and hence vasodilation. Presence of Bradykinin in excess amount is a possible reason for some of the side effects such as *dry cough and Angioedema* associated with ACE inhibitors.

ACEI and ARB **reduce blood pressure without affecting heart rate or cardiac output** because of their unique action in the peripheral vascular system. This feature is beneficial in patients with underlying bradycardia, hypotension or heart failure. They also have beneficial effect in preventing extensive remodeling of the myocardial smooth muscles after significant myocardial infarction or cardiomyopathy. Therefore, ACEI and ARBs play an integral part in treatment of patients post myocardial infarction and congestive heart failure.

Clinical use	Drug Category	Drug
Essential hypertension	ACEI	Captorpil, Benazepril, Enalapril, Quinapril, Fosinopril, Moexipril, Lisinopril, Perindopril, Ramipril, Trandalopril
	ARB	Losartan, Valsartan, Telmesartan,Olmesartan, Irbesartan, Candesartan, Eprosartan, Azilsartan
	Direct Renin Inhibitor	Aliskerin
Heart failure	ACEI	Captopril, Enalapril, Quinapril, Fosinopril, Moexipril, Lisinopril, Ramipril
	ARB	Valsartan, Candesatran
LV dysfunction after MI	ACEI	Captopril ,Lisinopril, Ramipril,Trandalopril
	ARB	Valsartan
Stroke reduction	ARB	Losartan
Diabetic nephropathy	ARB	Losartan,Irbesartan
	ACEI	Captopril
Asymptomatic LV dysfunction	ACEI	Enalapril

Table 5.4 Clinical use of specific RAAS drugs

Effect of ACEI and ARB

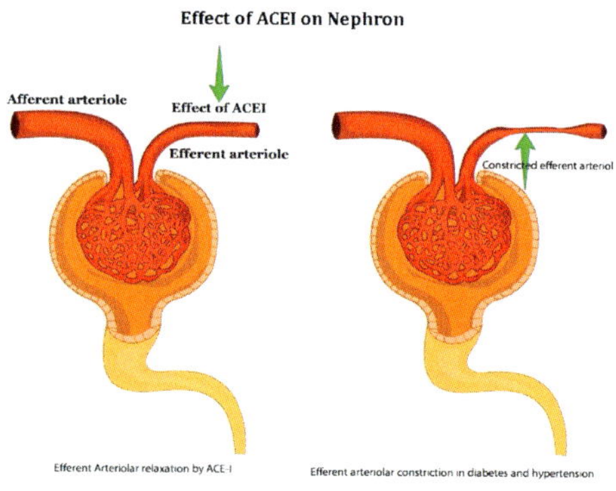

Fig 5.2 Effect of ACEI and ARB in renal arteries

ACEI and ARBs are generally used for the *protective effect on the renal system* in patients with hypertension and diabetes mellitus. In both cases, this group of medications cause *relaxation of* **efferent arterioles** of the glomerular system and thereby reduce intra glomerular capillary pressure. This reduction in pressure within the glomerular system improves renal hemodynamics and diminish proteinuria and glomerular hypertrophy. These actions slow down the rate of decline in GFR. They also **improve insulin sensitivity**, a beneficial factor in diabetes mellitus.

Adverse Reactions of ACEI and ARB

Dry cough is a common side-effect of ACEI, which is believed to be caused by increased amount of Bradykinin. The cough is generally absent in **Angiotensin receptor blockers** (ARB) as they do not affect Bradykinin synthesis and degradation. Interestingly, different agents in ACEI group produce symptoms of dry cough at various intensities. Therefore, changing from one agent to other within the same group can sometimes provide relief of symptoms.

Angioedema is a life-threatening side effect of ACEI, believed to be due to Bradykinin mechanism. Since it is a class effect for ACEI group of medications, *previous history of Angioedema is an absolute contraindication for use of ACEI*.

Both ACEI and ARBs are *contraindicated in* **bilateral renal artery stenosis.** In this condition, increased intravascular pressure as well as vasoconstriction is needed to maintain adequate renal perfusion. Vasodilation caused by these medications may result in acute renal tubular necrosis.

Contraindications of ACEI and ARB

- Bilateral renal artery stenosis
- Pregnancy
- Previous angioedema

Used with Caution

- Impaired renal function
- Elderly population
- Hypovolaemia and Hyponatraemia
- Hyperkalaemia (due to reduction in Aldosterone effect)

Points to remember!!!

- Renin- Angiotensin- Aldosterone system (RAAS) has a *predominant role in maintaining peripheral vascular resistance and systemic blood pressure*.

- Production of Renin is *stimulated by* factors such as *decreasing renal blood flow, hypotension, reduction in intravascular volume, sodium depletion* and *beta adrenergic stimulation*.

- Effects of RAAS is counterbalanced by the **Kallikrein- Kinin system**

- Primary effect of Bradykinin in the circulatory system is that of *vasodilatation* and *excretion of sodium* (Natriuresis). It also is an *inflammatory mediator*

- Presence of Bradykinin in excess amount is a possible reason for some of the side effects such as *dry cough and Angioedema* associated with ACE inhibitors

- ACEI and ARBs are generally used for their *protective effect on the renal system* in patients with hypertension and diabetes mellitus

- ACEI and ARBs also **improve insulin sensitivity** and is the beneficial factor in diabetes mellitus.

- Both ACEI and ARBs are *contraindicated in* **bilateral renal artery stenosis**

6 Diuretics

According to the eightth report of the Joint National committee on prevention, detection, evaluation, and treatment of high blood pressure (**JNC-8**) published by National Health Lung and blood Institute(NHLBI), **thiazide diuretic** is one of the *first line treatment* for management of *essential hypertension*. Depending on the mechanism and the site of action within the renal tubular system, diuretics can be classified into **Loop diuretics**, **Thiazide type diuretics**, **Potassium-sparing diuretics** and **Proximal tubular diuretics**. This classification and their examples are shown in the table.

Type	Site of action	Example
Proximal tubular diuretics (weak diuretics)	Proximal convoluted tubule	Acetazolamide Mannitol
Loop diuretics	Ascending loop of Henle	Furosemide Bumetanide Torsemide Ethacrynic acid
Thiazide diuretic	Distal convoluted tubule	Hydrochlorthiazide Methyclothiazide Chlorthalidone* Metolazone* Indapamide*
Potassium-sparing diuretics	Distal renal tubule	Amiloride Spironolactone Triamterene Eplerenone

* Sulfonamide compounds, used with caution in patients with sulfa allergy

Table 6.1 Classification of Diuretics

Mode of Action of Diuretics

Nephrons are the fundamental functional units of the kidney. There are about 0.8 to 1.5 million nephrons in an adult human kidney. They act as a regulatory mechanism for fluid and electrolyte balance of the body. Each nephron consists of *a filtration system* called **renal corpuscle** and a *reabsorption system* called

renal tubules. Renal corpuscle consists of a tuft of capillaries called **glomerulus** that receive blood from the renal arteries through **afferent** (towards) **arterioles**. The pressure within the renal arterial system force the fluid, electrolyte and other particles from the blood across the glomerular basement membrane into the space called **Bowman's capsules**. The fluid collected in the Bowman's capsules is known as **glomerular filtrate**. The blood drains out of the glomerular system through **efferent** (away) **arterioles,** which are *smaller in diameter than that of afferent arterioles*. This anatomic variation in the size of the arteries creates increased hydrostatic pressure within the glomerulus. This pressure is needed for pushing fluid and particles across the basement membrane.

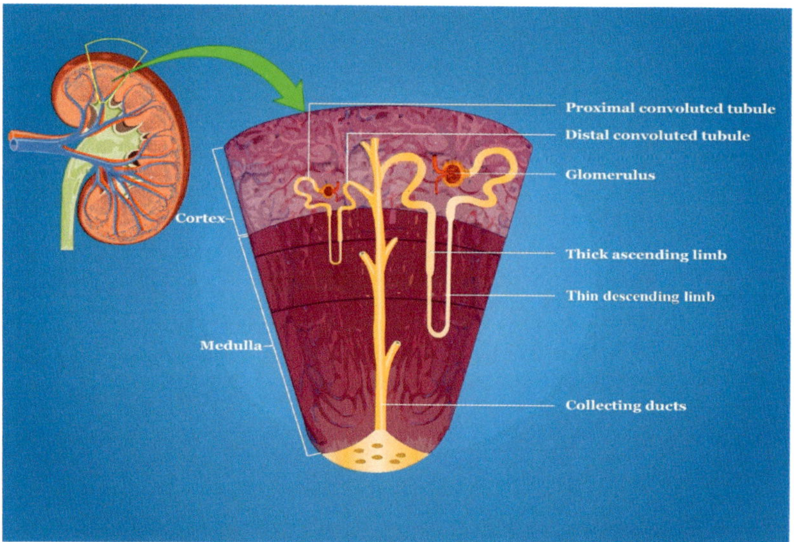

Fig 6.1 Structure of kidney and nephrons

The glomerular filtrate then moves through the renal tubules. During this movement, large quantity of particles and water are reabsorbed. Renal tubules consist of **proximal convoluted tubules**, **loop of Henle**, **distal convoluted tubules** and **collecting duct** system. Each part of this renal tubular system is lined with specialized cells capable of doing tubular secretion, excretion and reabsorption of various particles in to the glomerular filtrate. Each part of the renal tubule and its function is described in Fig. 6.2. The remaining urine flows into the renal papillae and then to the renal calyx from the collecting duct system. Subsequently, renal calyx drains into the renal pelvis which then connects to the ureter.

Functional Segments of Tubular System

Proximal tubule: This is the initial part of renal tubular system with characteristic **brush border cells** that increase surface area for absorption. *A large amount of glomerular filtrate including water*, *various salts* and *organic solutes* (*glucose and amino acid*) *are reabsorbed* back into the blood during this phase.

Loop of Henle : This is the long U-shaped segment of the renal tubular system. Loop of Henle is divided into **thin descending** and **thick ascending limb**. The **thin descending limb** is *permeable to water and impermeable to salts*. Nephrons with long thin descending loop help to reabsorb water and concentrate urine within the renal tubules. On the contrary, the **thick ascending loop** is *impermeable to water and actively involved in ion transport* through various countercurrents mechanism. This portion of the loop *actively pumps sodium out of the filtrate*.

Distal convoluted tubules : This part of the renal tubule involves in *active transport of various ions* and is predominantly regulated by endocrine system hormones ike **Aldosterone**, **Parathyroid hormone** etc.

Collecting duct system : This is the area of renal tubule where *majority of water reabsorption happens* because of the influence of **Anti Diuretic Hormone** (ADH). An increasing amount of ADH signals dehydration and therefore the kidney actively involves in conserving water by reabsorbing it from the glomerular filtrate back into the systemic circulation. For this purpose, ADH activates specialized membrane proteins called **Aquaporins** within the collecting duct system.

> Even though kidney constitutes less than 0.5% of total body weight, about 25% of cardiac output flows through the kidney in every minute (1.25 L/min).

The cells lining the renal tubule have their *one side exposed to the tubular fluid* (**apical membrane**) and the *other side to the blood vessels* (**Basolateral membrane**). Both of these membranes have various active and passive transport systems such as **Na^+-H^+ antiporter** (moving molecules in opposite direction), **Na^+-Phosphate symporter** (moving molecules in the same direction), **Na-K-ATPase**

pump etc. as illustrated in chapter 1. Sodium is reabsorbed in various parts of the renal tubule through specialized cells equipped with sodium transport mechanisms called **Na-K-ATPase pump**. These pumps perform the function by returning the reabsorbed sodium back in to the systemic circulation and maintain a low intra cellular sodium concentration. This in turn increases sodium and water losses, leading to beneficial effects of diuresis. Most of the pharmaceutical agents used as diuretics are acting by *interfering with Sodium reabsorption* at various levels of nephrons.

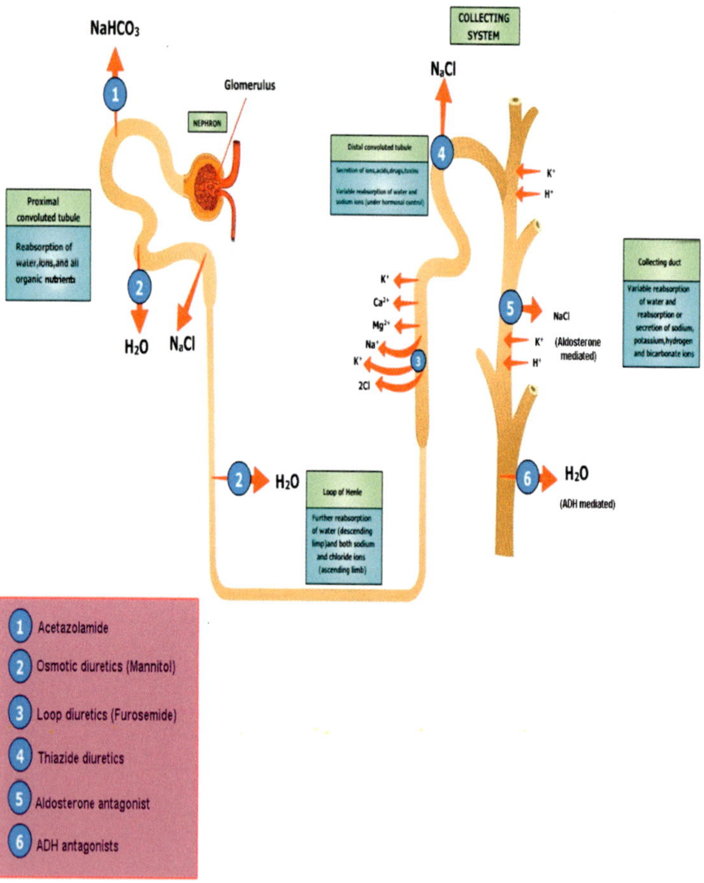

Fig 6.2 Action of diuterics at various parts of nephron

Loop diuretics act on **the ascending limb** of **Loop of Henle** and can cause *large amount of sodium excretion in a short duration of time*. However, **thiazide diuretics** are *weaker but long acting products that work in the* **distal convoluted tubules**. In the renal

The renal tubular system has the unique property of compensating for the loss of function of various proximal parts of the tubule by itself. For example, majority of sodium and water excretion happens in the proximal convoluted tubule; however, **Acetazolamide** that is a proximal tubular diuretic is not a strong diuretic agent. This is because *majority of water and sodium expelled from proximal tubule can be reabsorbed more distally in the system through compensatory mechanisms at the loop of Henle.*

Similar distal compensatory mechanism is seen in the action of loop diuretics where sodium and water expelled by the loop diuretics can be reabsorbed at the distal convoluted tubule. This is the rationale behind use of multiple agents like loop and thiazide diuretics together in treatment of refractory edema.

tubular system, up to 67% of sodium and water can be reabsorbed at the proximal convoluted tubule and 20% in the loop of Henle. Again, because of the compensatory mechanism, *loop diuretics work more effectively than proximal tubule diuretics*.

Loop diuretics like **Furosemide** works by *inhibiting the function of sodium potassium chloride transport mechanism in the apical membrane surface of the* **thick ascending limb of loop of Henle**. Loop diuretics compete with the chloride molecule within this transport system and thereby interfering the function of this transport mechanism. As an indirect result, *loop diuretics can affect* **calcium re-absorption** in the renal tubular system as *calcium is transported along with sodium* (co-transport) in this part of the tubule. This can cause loss of calcium through urine (**Calciuresis**) leading to renal calculi.

Beneficiary effect of diuretics in the treatment of hypertension can be traced to their property of **natriuresis** (urinary excretion of sodium) and thereby *reducing the amount of sodium in the vessel wall*. Since the contractile property of the artery is directly related to the amount of sodium in the arterial wall, presence of relatively small amounts of sodium facilitate dilation of peripheral cells and thereby reducing blood pressure. This in turn reduces the afterload of the heart and improves cardiac output.

Thiazide diuretics work at the **distal convoluted tubules** and can *inhibit the re-absorption of up to 5% of filtered sodium*. Since

Drug	Onset / peak	Half Life	Metabolism	Elimination
Loop diuretics				
Furosemide *Lasix®*	Oral 30 -60 min IV less than 5 min	0.5-2 hrs Up to 9 hrs (renal disease)	Minimal hepatic	Urine, Feces
Bumetanide *Bumex®*	Oral 30 to 60 min IV 2 to 3 min	1 to 1.5 hrs	Partially hepatic	Urine
Torsemide *Demadex®*	Within 1 hr	3.5 hrs	Hepatic	Urine
Ethacrynic acid *Edecrin®*	Oral 30 min IV 5 min	2-4 hrs	Hepatic	Feces and urine
Thiazide type diuretics				
Chlorthalidone *Thalitone®*	2 to 6 hours	40 to 60 hrs	Hepatic	Urine
Hydrochlorothiazide *Microzide®*	Less than 2 hours	5 to 14 hrs	Not metabolized	Urine
Metolazone *Zaroxolyn®*	One hour	20 hrs	Minimal	Urine
Indapamide *Lozol®*	2 hours	14 to 25 hrs	Extensive hepatic	Urine
Potassium-sparing diuretics				
Amiloride *Midamor®*	2 hours 8-144 hrs (renal failure)	6-9 hrs	Not metabolized	Urine, feces
Spironolactone *Aldactone®*	3-4 hours	1.3-2 hrs (Spironolactone) 10 to 23 hrs (Canrenone*)	hepatic	urine, feces
Triamterene *Dyrenium®*	2 to 4 hours	3 hrs	Hepatic	Urine
Proximal tubular diuretics				
Acetazolamide *Diamox®*	Oral 2 hrs IV 10 min	10- 15 hrs	None	Urine
Osmotic diuretic				
Mannitol *Osmitrol®*	1- 3 hrs	4.5 hrs	Minimal hepatic	Urine
Vasopressin receptor antagonist				
Tolvaptan** *Samsca®*	2-4 hrs	5-12 hrs	Hepatic	Feces
Conivaptan *Vaprisol®*	12 hrs (peak)	5-8 hrs	Hepatic	Feces and Urine

* Active metabolite, ** Used for treatment of hyponatremia

Table 6.2 Pharmacokinetics of major diuretics

Clinical use	Drug Category	Drug
Edema	Thiazide diuretic	Chlorthalidone Hydrochlorothiazide Indapamide Metolazone
	Loop diuretics	Furosemide Bumetanide
	Potassium-sparing diuretics	Amiloride Spironolactone Triamterene
	Proximal tubular diuretics	Acetazolamide
Hypertension	Thiazide diuretic	Chlorthalidone Hydrochlorothiazide Indapamide Metolazone(adjunct)
	Loop diuretics	Furosemide
	Potassium-sparing diuretic	Amiloride Spironolactone Triamterene
Refractory edema	Thiazide diuretic	Metolazone
	Loop diuretics	Furosemide Bumetanide
Congestive heart failure	Potassium-sparing diuretic	Spironolactone*
Glaucoma, Altitude sickness, Seizure	Proximal tubular diuretic	Acetazolamide

* Due to Aldosterone modulator effect

Table 6.3.Clinical use of major diuretics

there is only a small amount of sodium reabsorbed in this segment of the tubule, *thiazide diuretics by nature are weak diuretics*.

Potassium-sparing diuretics work in the **collecting duct system** by influencing **Aldosterone sensitive sodium channels** in this area. *Naturally occurring sodium reabsorption in this part of the tubule facilitates potassium excretion.* Therefore, inhibition of sodium reabsorption results in excessive accumulation of potassium leading to **hyperkalemia**. **Canrenone** is one of the active metabolite of **Spironolactone,** which is actively involved in the pharmacologic effects of this drug.

Proximal convoluted tubular diuretics like **Acetazolamide** provides natriuresis and diuresis by *inhibiting the activity of carbonic unhydrase*. This is a week diuretic compared to the other agents because of the compensatory reabsorption of sodium and water in the distal aspect of the tubular system.

Vasopressin receptor antagonists are used in facilitating *selective water diuresis by inhibiting antidiuretic hormone receptors*. More than for treatment of edema, these agents are used in management of **hyponatremia** in which excessive water loss facilitated by these agents in turn produces effective hypernatremia. Examples are **Tolvaptan** and **Conivaptan.**

Mannitol is an osmotic diuretic that *inhibits sodium and water reabsorption in both proximal tubule and loop of Henle*. Mannitol produces osmotic diuresis by increasing the osmotic pressure of glomerular filtrate, which inhibits tubular reabsorption of water and electrolytes, hence increases urinary output. Another major effect of Mannitol compared to other diuretics is its *ability to facilitate water loss without significant sodium and potassium excretion*. This preferential water loss induced by mannitol can lead to hypovolemia and hypernatremia with repeated application.

Points to remember!!!

- **According to JNC 8 thiazide diuretics** is one of the first line treatment for management of *essential hypertension*.
- Each nephron consists of *a filtration system* called **renal corpuscle** and a *reabsorption system* called **renal tubules**.
- **Proximal tubule** is the initial part of renal tubular system with characteristic **brush border cells** that increase surface area for absorption.
- *A large amount of glomerular filtrate including water, various salts* and *organic solutes* (*glucose and amino acid*) *are reabsorbed* back into the blood at **Proximal tubule**
- Loop of Henle is divided into **thin descending** and **thick ascending limb**.
- The **thin descending limb** is *permeable to water and impermeable to salts*.
- The **thick ascending loop** is *impermeable to water and actively involved in ion transport* through various countercurrents mechanism.
- **Distal convoluted tubules** involve in *active transport of various*

ions and are regulated by endocrine system hormones such as **Aldosterone**, **Parathyroid hormone** etc.

- **Collecting duct system** is the area of renal tubule where *majority of water reabsorption happens* because of the influence of **Anti Diuretic Hormone**

- Most of the pharmaceutical agents used as diuretics are acting by *interfering with Sodium reabsorption* at various levels of nephrons.

- **Loop diuretics** acts on **the ascending limb** of **Loop of Henle** and can cause *large amount of sodium excretion in a short duration of time.*

- **Thiazide diuretics** are *weaker but long acting products that work in the* **distal convoluted tubules**.

- **Furosemide** acts by *inhibiting the function of sodium potassium chloride transporting mechanism in the apical membrane surface of the* **thick ascending limb of loop of Henle**.

- *Loop diuretics can affect* **calcium reabsorption** in the renal tubular system leading to renal calculi

- **Thiazide diuretics** work at the **distal convoluted tubules** and can *inhibit the reabsorption of up to 5% of filtered sodium.*

- **Potassium-sparing diuretics** work in the **collecting duct system** by influencing **Aldosterone sensitive sodium channels**

- Inhibition of sodium reabsorption by potassium sparing diuretics results in excessive accumulation of potassium leading to **hyperkalemia**.

- **Proximal convoluted tubular diuretics** like **Acetazolamide** provides natriuresis and diuresis by *inhibiting the activity of carbonic unhydrase.*

- **Mannitol** is an osmotic diuretic which *inhibits sodium and water reabsorption in both proximal tubule as well as the loop of Henle.*

- Mannitol has *ability to facilitate water loss without significant sodium and potassium excretion.*

7 Antiplatelets and Anticoagulants

Antiplatelets and anticoagulants are one of the mainstay pharmacologic agents used in cardiovascular care. They range from the common antiplatelet Aspirin to the recombinant Tissue Plasminogen Activator (rTPA) used for thrombolysis in myocardial infarction. In order to better understand the mechanism of action and clinical effect of various agents, it is important to recognize the basics of hematopoiesis, coagulation and bleeding.

Components of the Blood

The most important function of circulating blood is to carry oxygen and nutrients to the tissue and remove carbon dioxide and other waste products. Circulating blood also involves in transferring chemicals such as hormones and drugs to the target receptor sites. Based on the presence of antigen and antibody, there are distinct blood groups identified and that helps in assessing compatibility between individuals as shown in the table.

Blood group	Antigen	Antibody	Compatibility
Group A	Antigen A	Antibodies to B	Group A, Group O
Group B	Antigen B	Antibodies to A	Group B, Group O
Group A-B	Both antigen A and B	No antibodies	**Universal recipient**
Group O	No antigen	Antibodies to A, B	**Universal donor**

Table 7.1 Common blood groups

Major components of blood are **red blood cells** (Erythrocytes), **white blood cells** (Leukocytes) and **platelets** (Thrombocytes) suspended in a complex carrier solution called **plasma**.

Erythrocytes: They are *flexible biconcave disc shaped cells without a nucleus and contain* **hemoglobin**. They originate from the stem cells in the bone marrow. Production of erythrocytes (Erythropoiesis) is regulated by a substance called **Erythropoietin**

released from the kidney.

Leukocytes: White blood cells include **Granulocytes** (65%), **Lymphocytes** (30%) and **Monocytes** (5%). **Granulocytes** are further divided into **Neutrophils** (95%), **Eosinophils** (4%) and **Basophils** (1%). Among leukocytes, ***Granulocytes** and **Monocytes** are actively involved in defending the body against microbes* by attacking and engulfing foreign objects (**phagocytosis**). The ***lymphocytes** produce humoral and cell mediated immunity* through B-lymphocytes and T-lymphocytes.

Platelets: Platelets are essentially *cell fragments produced from disintegration of* **megakaryocytes**. The production of platelets are regulated by a substance called **Thrombopoietin**. They are an essential component in the process of hemostasis by adhering to the damaged blood vessels wall and *provide both mechanical barrier and a platform for further coagulation process*. They also release various chemicals like **Adenosine Diphosphate** (ADP) and **Thromboxane A_2** through the use of **Cyclooxygenase enzyme.** This enzyme attracts other platelets and coagulation components to the site of injury to facilitate blood clotting.

> Aspirin induces its anti-platelet function by interfering with Cyclooxygenase pathway during platelet aggregation. NSAID also have the same effect and is the reason behind antiplatelet effect of these agents. Clopidogrel, Ticlopidine and Prasugrel acts by inhibiting ADP pathway.

Platelets also release **Serotonin** at the time of injury that *causes localized vasoconstriction*. Another product called **Thromboplastin** released from platelets accelerates blood coagulation process. Along with **Thromboxane A_2**, platelets release the prostaglandin named **Prostacyclin I_2** (PGI_2). This product *causes vasodilation and inhibition of platelet adherence*. Careful balancing of these counteracting products in the platelet aggregation mechanism *limits clotting process to only at the site of injury* and avoid clotting from happening elsewhere in the vessel.

Coagulation Process

This is the final process by which hemostasis is attained after bleeding. In response to a vessel injury, platelets are aggregated at the site of damage and start creating a temporary plug on the vessel wall. The *bond between platelets and the injured vessel wall* (***platelet adherence***) is ensured by **von Willebrand factor** (**vWF**) that acts as a bridge between platelets and vessel wall. Because of the effect of **Thromboxane A_2** as mentioned earlier, more platelets are subsequently adhered to provide considerable mechanical barrier. **Calcium ions** also play a major role in platelet aggregation. **Thromboxane A_2** also facilitates activation of **glycoprotein IIb/IIIa receptors** on the platelet surface, which in turn *exposes fibrinogen binding sites on the platelet surface*. By this mechanism, loosely held aggregates of platelets are bound together to create more stable mass.

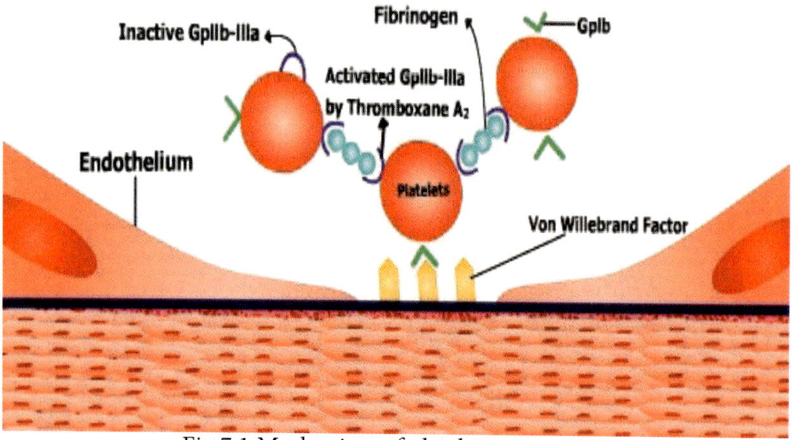

Fig 7.1 Mechanism of platelet aggregation

The final phase of the formation of **fibrin clot** happens through a complex process with a series of enzymatic reactions and sequential activation of otherwise inactive clotting factors. This process is known as **coagulation cascade**. This pathway can be initiated by two different mechanisms called **Extrinsic pathway** (**tissue pathway**) and **Intrinsic pathway**. After a series of enzymatic activation, both of these pathways come down to a common series of chemical processes known as **common pathway**. Detailed description of coagulation pathway is explained in Fig 7.2.

There are 12 different clotting factors as shown in the box.

Coagulation Factors	
Factor I	Fibrinogen
Factor II	Prothrombin
Factor III	Tissue factor (Thromboplastin)
Factor IV	Calcium
Factor V	Labile factor (Accelerator Globulin)
Factor VII	Stable factor (Serum Prothrombin Conversion Accelerator (SPCA))
Factor VIII	Anti hemophilic factor A
Factor IX	Christmas factor (Anti hemophilic factor B)
Factor X	Stuart factor (Thrombokinase or Power factor)
Factor XI	Plasma Thromboplastin Antecedent (PTA) (Anti hemophilic factor C)
Factor XII	Hageman factor (Anti hemophilic factor D)
Factor XIII	Fibrin stabilizing factor (FSF)

Box 7.1Coagulation factors

Fibrinolysis

Fibrinolysis is the *enzymatic degradation of fibrin clot after the vessel injury is stabilized*. This process is carried out mainly by the enzyme called **Plasmin**. **Plasminogen** is the precursor of active plasmin and is synthesized in the liver. Even though plasminogen is not capable of degrading fibrin by itself, it has a great affinity for fibrin and is incorporated into the blood clots when they are formed.

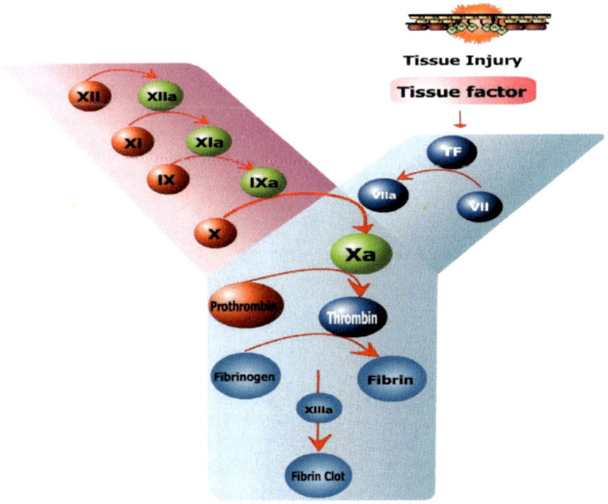

Table 7.2 Coagulation and anticoagulation pathways

Laboratory Measurements of Coagulation			
Laboratory test	**Clotting pathway**	**Normal Value**	**Clinical Use**
Activated Partial Thromboplastin Time (**aPTT**)	Analyze **Intrinsic pathway**	21-35 Sec*	Increased with Heparin or Thrombin inhibitor therapy
Prothrombin time (**PT**)	Analyze extrinsic pathway (**Tissue pathway**)	11-13 Sec*	Increase with liver disease, Coumadin therapy, Vitamin K deficiency, Factor VII, X, II, V or I deficiency
Thrombin time	Analyzes **Common pathway**	<20Sec*	Increased in fibrinolytic therapy, Heparin, Hirudin, Multiple myeloma, low fibrinogen levels, DIC, liver disease, increased fibrin degradation protein (FDP)
International Normalized Ratio (**INR**)	For standardization of PT measurements	0.8-1.2 (No specific units since it is a ratio)	Increase with liver disease, Coumadin therapy, Vitamin K deficiency, Factor VII, X, II, V or I deficiency
Bleeding time(**BT**)	Rate of platelet adhesion and aggregation	3-10 min	Increased in platelet abnormalities, antiplatelet therapy, liver disease
Protein C	Effectiveness of natural anticoagulation	4-5 μ g/ml	For hypercoagulable disorders
D-dimer (a FDP)	The level of endogenous fibrinolysis	<400 ng/ml	Elevated in excessive endogenous clotting such as DVT, PE, DIC**
Activated clotting time (ACT)	To determine effectiveness of heparin	70-120 sec	Increased with Heparin and reduced with Protamine Sulfate
Fibrin Degradation Protein(FDP)	Fibrinolysis process	<10 μg/ml	Elevated in DIC, liver disease and fibrinolysis

* Depending on the laboratory; **DVT- Deep Vein Thrombosis, PE- Pulmonary Embolus, DIC- Disseminated Intravascular Coagulation

Table 7.2 Laboratory measurements of coagulation

Tissue plasminogen activator (**t-PA**) and **Urokinase** *facilitate conversion of plasminogen to plasmin and thereby fibrinolysis*. When the fibrin clot is broken down, it's fragments known as **fibrin degradation products** (**FDP**) are released into the circulation. They themselves *act as potent anticoagulants*.

Natural Anticoagulation

Under normal circumstances, *unwanted coagulation process in the body is inhibited by a naturally occurring anticoagulation system* consists of **Antithrombin III**, **Heparin cofactor II**, **Protein C** and **Protein S**. Coagulation abnormalities are prevented by *maintaining a balance between the amount of activated clotting factors*, *inhibitors of coagulation and degradation of fibrin clot*. Among these agents, **Antithrombin III** is considered as a major inhibitor of coagulation. It slowly *inactivates active forms of clotting factors X*, *IX*, *XI*, *XII* and *thrombin*. **Heparin cofactor II** inhibits both **Thrombin** and **Thrombin induced platelet aggregation**. *Functions of both of these factors are greatly increased in the presence of*

Heparin.

Protein C is a vitamin K dependent protein, synthesized in the liver and is circulated in the blood in its inactive form. When combined with **Thrombin**, Protein C is activated to form activated protein C (**APC**), which in *turn inactivates* Factor V_a and Factor VIII_a. Protein C also promotes fibrinolysis by *inactivating inhibitors of t-PA* and thereby *facilitating conversion of plasminogen to plasmin*. **Protein S** is also a vitamin K dependent glycoprotein synthesized in the endothelium. This substance acts as a cofactor for Protein C in *inactivation of* factor V_a and factor VIII_a.

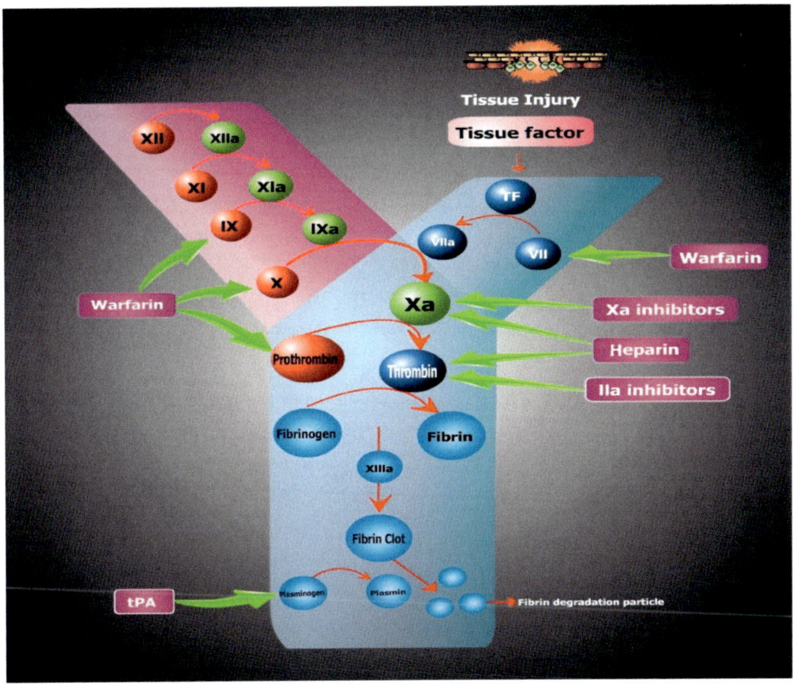

Fig 7.3 Site of action of anticoagulants in cloating cascade

Anticoagulants

Anticoagulants are the cornerstone in management of not only cardiac conditions, but also other vascular pathologies ike venous thrombosis and stroke. They are available in both oral and parenteral forms. Commonly, parenteral anticoagulants are reserved for acute care settings whereas long-term management is achieved through their oral counterparts.

Unfractionated Heparin (UFH)

This type of heparin acts as an anticoagulants by augmenting *the inhibitory function of* **Antithrombin III** on clotting **factor II** (**Thrombin**), **XII**, **XI**, **IX** and **factor Xa**. It also *prevents the formation of a stable clot by inhibiting* **fibrin stabilizing factor** (**factor XIII**). Unfractionated heparin is a very large molecule with average molecular weight upwards of **15,000 Da** (Dalton unit). Because of its *large structure*, *unfractionated heparin can attach to both **Thrombin** and **factor Xa*** whereas other derivatives of heparin with small molecular structure like **low molecule weight heparin** (**LMWH**) *can only inhibit factor Xa*. UFH is administered parenterally as it cannot be absorbed from the GI tract.

UFH has *immediate onset of action when given intravenously*. The clinical effect varies from patient to patient because of high protein binding. It is metabolized by the liver and excreted through the kidneys. UFH has high *affinity for plasma proteins and other cellular components* in the blood. This affinity *causes lower therapeutic benefits and increased chance of immunologic reaction* like **heparin induced thrombocytopenia** (**HIT**). It also has a non-linear dose response approach in which a *small change in dosage can lead to large effect in anticoagulation response*. Adequacy of treatment with unfractionated heparin can be monitored by doing **activated Partial Thromboplastin Time** (**aPTT**). Major adverse effect of heparin therapy is bleeding complications. Thrombocytopenia and osteoporosis are commonly seen with long-term treatments.

Heparin Induced Thrombocytopenia (HIT)

This disorder is usually seen in patients undergoing *prolonged treatment* (*>4 days*) using heparin. There are two types of heparin induced thrombocytopenia. The **type I** (benign form) is caused by **platelet sequestration**, usually happens in the beginning of the treatment. In this situation, the *platelet count rarely goes less than 100,000/mm^3*. Type I Heparin induced thrombocytopenia usually *resolves without any intervention and is clinically insignificant*.

The second form of heparin induced thrombocytopenia is **immune-mediated** with the *onset of symptoms from 5 to 15 days after heparin administration*. Earlier than five days of onset is seen in patients who were exposed to heparin within 1 to 2 months prior to the current episode. **Type II heparin induced thrombocytopenia** (**HIT-II**) is also called **White clot syndrome** because of the *presence of platelet rich arterial thrombus more than fibrin rich venous thrombus*. Platelet count *less than 100,000/ mm^3 or less than 50% of the baseline* is common in this form of disease. Here, an IgG mediated immune reaction leads to the formation of antibodies against the **heparin-platelet factor 4 complexes** (**PF4**). *Widespread platelet activation and subsequent aggregation* result in arterial and venous thrombosis causing limb ischemia, myocardial infarction, deep vein thrombosis, pulmonary embolism etc.

Immediate discontinuation of all heparin sources including heparin flushes is required until platelet count normalizes. Even though theoretically low molecule weight heparin (LMWH) products are possible alternative in HIT, cross sensitivity between unfractionated and low molecule weight heparin prevents the use of even LMWH in this situation. Other approved agents for treatment of patients with the HIT are **Bivalirudin** (**Angiomax®**), **Argatroban** (both are *direct thrombin inhibitors*), **Fondaparinux** (**Arixtra®**- a *factor Xa inhibitor*) and **Lepirudin** (*recombinant Hirudin*). In the absence of bleeding, all patients with heparin induced thrombocytopenia should be treated with alternate anticoagulants because of the high risk of further thrombosis. In long-term, these patients are transitioned into oral anticoagulants like warfarin when the platelets are regained and are adequately anticoagulated with above-mentioned agents.

Low Molecular Weight Heparin (LMWH)

This type of heparin is produced by *controlled enzymatic depolymerization of unfractionated heparin* (UFH) *that results in smaller low molecular weight fragments*. They generally have a mean molecule weight of **5000 Da units**. Homogeneous nature of LMWH helps to avoid many of the practical hurdles that unfractionated heparin has in the real world. However, the smaller structure makes them having less affinity to the thrombin and therefore LMWH attains its *anticoagulation effect through* **antithrombin III** *activation and resulting* **factor X a** *inhibition*. Because of the less affinity to plasma proteins and other cellular material compared to that of unfractionated heparin, *LMWH has better pharmacologic profiles with a predictable action from patient to patient*. This predictability helps in avoiding subsequent routine

Advantageous of LMWH over UFH

- Greater bioavailability
- Longer duration of action
- Predictable anticoagulation response
- Easy dosing because of anticoagulation response directly related to body weight
- Less chance of heparin induced thrombocytopenia
- Lower risk of osteoporosis
- Safer for outpatient administration

Box 7.2 Advantages of LMWH over UFH

laboratory monitoring unlike in the case of UFH. They also have longer half-life in the plasma compared to that of unfractionated heparin. Because of its *renal clearance* for excretion, LMWH can be accumulated in patients with renal disease. Compared to the 30% bioavailability with unfractionated heparin, LMWH has *90% bioavailability* that provides better performance.

Synthetic Low Molecule Weight Heparin

A synthetic form of low molecule weight heparin, **antithrombin binding pentasaccharide** sequence called **Fondaparinux** (**Arixtra**®) differ from both unfractionated heparin and regular low molecule weight heparin in terms of its substantially low molecule weight of **1728** Dalton unit. Because of the short chain nature, it only attaches to antithrombin III and subsequently

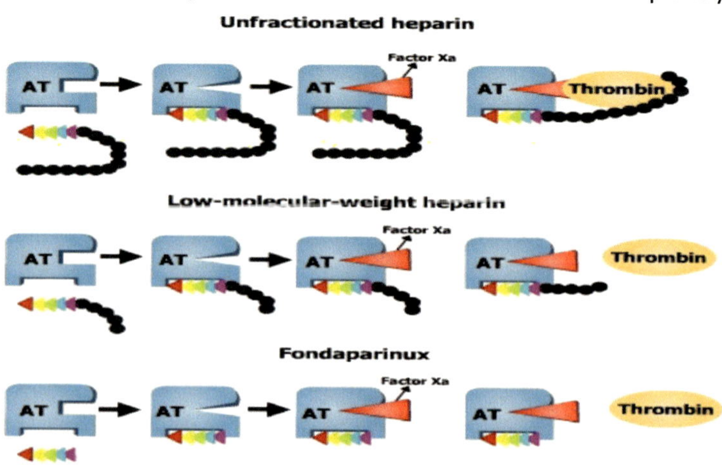

Fig 7.4 Mechanism of action of UFH, LMWH and Fondaparinux

get anticoagulation effect primarily through factor Xa inhibition without affecting thrombin. They provide *100% bioavailability* after subcutaneous injection and provide predictable anticoagulation response.

Direct Thrombin Inhibitors

Unlike unfractionated heparin and low molecule weight heparin using antithrombin III as a cofactor to inhibit thrombin, **direct thrombin inhibitors** *target* **thrombin** *molecule itself to achieve their anticoagulation effect*. They are available in both IV and Oral preparations. Common examples of IV preparations are are **Lepirudin**, **Argatroban**, **Bivalirudin** and **Desirudin**. Oral Factor Xa inhibitors are collectively known as **Noval Oral Anticoaguant** agents (NOAC). **Dabigatran**(Pradaxa®), **Rivaroxaban** (Xarelto®) and **Apixaban** (Eliquis®),**Edoxaban** (Savaysa®), and **Betrixaban** (Bevyxxa®) are currently available in the market for indications ranging from treatment of non valvular atrial fibrillation to venous thromboembolism (VTE) prophylaxis.

The *most important clinical advantage of using direct thrombin inhibitors* over other forms of heparin *are their ability to inactivate the thrombin bound to the clot*. Contrary to the action of heparin and low molecule weight heparin, these agents *do not interact with* **platelet factor (PF4)** which is responsible for **heparin induced thrombocytopenia**. Therefore, both *Lepirudin* and *Argatroban are approved for treatment of HIT*. Among these,

Comparison of Different Direct Thrombin Inhibitors

	Hirudin	Bivalirudin	Argatroban	Dabigatran
Route	IV	IV	IV	PO
Plasma half-life	60 min	25 min	45	12 to 17 hours
Excretion	renal	renal	hepatic	Renal
Monitoring	aPTT	aPTT*	aPTT	aPTT**
Uses	`not available HIT	HIT PCI	HIT	non-valvular atrial fibrillation (Stroke prophylaxis)

* Practically not needed because of short half-life

**clinically not indicated

Table 7.3.Comparison between Direct thrombin Inhibitors

Lepirudin is no longer available in the US market as of the beginning of 2013.

Bivalirudin (**Angiomax®**) is a *synthetic analogue of* ***Hirudin*** among direct thrombin inhibitor group. It is commonly *used for anticoagulation during* **percutaneous coronary intervention**. Its plasma half-life of **25 min** coupled with low incidence of abnormal bleeding made the drug an attractive choice over other heparin products for this purpose. Like many other anticoagulants, Bivalirudin has a **renal excretion process** and therefore *used with caution in patients with renal insufficiency*. It can also be used for *anticoagulation in patients with heparin induced thrombocytopenia*.

Thrombolytics

Fibrinolytics play a major role in chemical revascularization of patients with acute myocardial infarction and stroke. Even though percutaneous catheter-based mechanical revascularization (PCI) or thrombectomy are the mainstay treatment choices If available, treatment with fibrinolytics to meet "**door to needle**" time for appropriate patients is still in use. Selection criteria for patients undergoing thrombolytic therapy in myocardial infarction/acute

Contraindications for Fibrinolytic Therapy
Absolute contraindications • History of intracranial hemorrhage • Known intracranial neoplasm or AV malformation • Ischemic stroke within last three months(except current episode) • Active bleeding disorders excluding menstruation • Significant closed head or facial trauma within last three months
Relative contraindication • History of poorly controlled malignant hypertension (SBP>180) • Severe uncontrolled hypertension upon presentation (SBP>180, DBP>110) • Dementia or other intracranial pathology • History of stroke greater than three months ago • Recent internal bleeding (within 2 to 4 weeks) • Traumatic or prolonged CPR (greater than 10 min) • Major surgery (less than three weeks) • Non-compressible bleeding • Pregnancy • Active peptic ulcer • Current use of other anticoagulants • Prior allergic reactions (especially for Streptokinase)

Box 7.3 Selection criteria for Fibrinolytic therapy

Name	Trade name	Uses
Streptokinase	Streptase® *	Acute myocardial infarction, pulmonary embolism
Urokinase	Kinlytic®*	Massive pulmonary embolism
Alteplase (t-PA)	Activase® Cathflo® Activase®	STEMI, acute PE, acute ischemic stroke Central venous catheter clearance
Tenectaplace	TNKase	STEMI**
Reteplace	Retavase®	STEMI**

* Not available in US

** it is recommended that all patients receiving these agents should get 162 to 325 mg of chewable non coated Aspirin as soon as possible an concurrent heparin 60 units/kg bolus (max 4000 Units) with infusion of 12 Units/kg/hr)

Table 7.4 Fibrinolytic agents

stroke are given in box 7.4.

All of the fibrinolytics agents are performing their action through *conversion of* **plasminogen** *to active* **plasmin**. Under normal circumstances, plasminogen can be seen in two different forms, as circulating plasminogen and that bound to the fibrin clot. Currently available fibrinolytics agents can be classified into two categories based on their specificity for the fibrin bound plasminogen. **First generation fibrinolytic agents** such as **Streptokinase**, **Anistreplace**

Criteria for Treatment with Fibrinolytics

Acute ST elevation myocardial infarction

- Chest pain ≥ 20min
- Onset of chest pain within last 12 hours
- Onset of chest pain within 12 to 24 hours with ischemic symptoms
- ST elevation >0.1mV in at least two contiguous* leads
- New or presumably new Left bundle Branch Block (LBBB)

Acute stroke

- Onset of symptoms within three hours

Acute pulmonary embolism

- Documented massive pulmonary embolism
  (PE with hypotension i.e. SBP< 90 or on inotropic support)
- Age ≤75 yrs
- Persistent profound bradycardia
- Severe right ventricular dysfunction

* Two leads looking at the same or neighboring anatomical areas of the heart. For e g. lead II and III for inferior wall of myocardium.

Box 7.4 Treatment criteria for Fibrinolytic therapy

and **Urokinase** are *non-specific for fibrin bound plasminogen* and therefore affect both pools of plasminogen resulting in a generalized effect.

However, the newer generation of **recombinant tissue plasminogen activator** (**rt-PA**) agents such as **Alteplase** or **Activase**, and its derivatives **Tenecteplase** (**TNKase®**) and **Reteplase** (**Retavase®**) are *fibrin bound plasminogen specific* and has a better clinical benefit.

Streptokinase produces *hypotension* and has *immune-mediated effects* that cause *antibody production resulting in possible allergic reactions*. These side effects are absent in recombinant agents. Recommended criteria for treatment with fibrinolytic agents during myocardial infarction, pulmonary embolism and acute stroke are detailed in the box.

Vitamin K Antagonists

One of the major **vitamin K antagonist** widely used in clinical practice is **Coumadin** (**Warfarin**). It was originally derived from a group of compounds used as rodent killers in 1950s. These rodenticides were exerting their lethal effect by causing severe hemorrhage in their intended victims. The drug **Coumadin** used for therapeutic purposes in human being has much less potency than its above-mentioned counterparts. Coumadin achieves the anticoagulation effect through *inhibiting activation of* **vitamin K dependent** *clotting factors such as* **factor II**, **VII**, **IX** *and* **X**. It *also affects anticoagulants factors such as* **Protein C** and **Protein S**. For prevention of clotting, Coumadin work through **extrinsic pathway** of clotting cascade. Coumadin *interferes with the activation of inactive vitamin K into its active form*. It has a half-life of **36 to 42** hours.

Even though Coumadin affect above-mentioned clotting

Patients in hypercoagulable state (e.g. pulmonary embolism), Coumadin should not be initiated *without concurrent use of another anticoagulants* like **Enoxaparin** *in order to avoid thrombosis in the initial phase* of treatment. This happens because, along with depletion of vitamin K dependent clotting factors, Coumadin also *cause drop in natural anticoagulation factors* such as **Protein C** and **Factor II**. Lack of these anticoagulation factors create a paradoxical hypercoagulable situation until therapeutic level of Coumadin is achieved.

The PT measurements of a healthy individual can vary from place to place depending on the variation between different batches of tissue factor in the reagent and the analytical system used. **International Normalized Ratio** (INR) is devised to standardize the **Prothrombin time (PT)** values obtained from laboratory reagents with varying sensitivity across the world. In order to standardize this process, each reagent is compared against an international reference tissue factor and given a sensitivity index(ISI). INR is calculated by the ratio of patient's Prothrombin time to the control sample raised to the power of International Sensitivity Index (ISI) for the particular reagent-system combination.

factors, it is worth noting that *coumadin does not inactivate existing clotting factors* in the blood. This explains the reason behind **delayed onset of the therapeutic action** by Coumadin. When administered, clotting factors with shorter half-life such as **factor VII** (half-life 6 hrs) depletes early on. However, **factor II** which has a half-life of 60 hours remains active. Therefore, *effective therapeutic action of Coumadin in the blood is achieved after an average of three days (72 hrs) from the time of initial dose*.

Presence of heparin in the blood sample can result in **falsely elevated INR**. In day-to-day clinical practice, this error can be avoided by collecting blood from peripheral veins rather than from a central venous catheter that could be contaminated with heparin.

Moreover, there are many other factors ranging from genetic variations to the type of diet the patient follows may

Factors Affecting INR in Coumadin Therapy

Increases INR	Reduce INR
• Genetic variation (CYP2C9) • Hepatic disease, CHF • Alcohol abuse • Vitamin K deficiency • Febrile illness & hypothyroidism (hypo metabolic state)* • Medications • Food items (Ginger, Garlic, Turmeric)	• Dietary changes in Vitamin K intake(Greens, Avocado, Green tea) • Intake of Vitamin K supplements (Multivitamins, herbal products) • Disease state (Hyperthyroidism, fat mal-absorption) • Smoking (contains Vit K)

*cause depletion of vitamin K

Table 7.5 Factors affecting INR

influence therapeutic anticoagulation by Coumadin. Because of its very narrow therapeutic window, this drug should be monitored closely in order to prevent bleeding complications from toxicity and thromboembolism from inadequate dosage. Effectiveness of anticoagulation with Coumadin is monitored through **Prothrombin** and **International normalized ratio (INR)**. For practical purposes INR is more suitable for assessing adequacy of dosage.

Medications and Food Items Influence Coumadin

Potentiating factors	Inhibiting factors
• Alcohol • Amiodarone • Steroids • Antibiotics (Erythromycin, Metronidazole, Bactrim) • Antifungal • Salicylate • NSAIDs • H_2 antagonist and PPI (Cimetidine, Omeprazole) • Thyroid hormones • Anticonvulsants • Anti-lipidemic agents • Flu vaccine	• High vitamin K containing food (greens) • Anti-thyroid medication • Bile acid sequestrants • Carbamazepine • Coenzyme Q-10 • Some oral contraceptives

Table 7.6 Medications and food items influence Coumadin

Coumadin *binds extensively with plasma proteins* and therefore only a small fraction of the drug administered is actually available for biologic functions. This feature along with a narrow therapeutic window of Coumadin makes it very sensitive in terms of managing individual patient's dosage. *Patients at high risk for bleeding include elderly clients*, *patients with congestive heart failure*, *underlying malignancy*, *severely impaired hepatic or renal dysfunction*, *inadequate nutrition*, *previous history of GI bleeding* etc. These group of patients should receive a lower initial dose to prevent bleeding complications.

Many of the common food items, especially **green leafy vegetables** affects therapeutic effect of Coumadin because of *the high vitamin K content*. Common examples of high vitamin K containing food items are Chinese green tea (1428 μg/100 gm), cooked coriander or cilantro leaves (1510 μg / 100 gm). Raw lettuce, spinach and broccoli contain an average of 200-300 μg of Vit K/100gm serving. Patients with a high thromboembolic risk on Coumadin should avoid these food items to prevent inconsistencies in their therapeutic anticoagulation.

Treatment of Supratherapeutic INR Secondary to Coumadin Toxicity	
INR<5 without bleeding	• Withhold next dose and reduce subsequent dosage • Evaluate INR in 7-14 days • Modify the underlying factor*
INR 5 to 9 without bleeding	• Withhold next 1-2 doses of Coumadin and give oral vitamin K (2.5 mg) • Re-evaluate INR in 24-48 hrs • Modify the underlying factor*
INR >9 without bleeding	• Withhold Coumadin and give oral vitamin K (2.5 to 5 mg) • Re evaluate INR in 24 Hrs • Modify the underlying factor*
Elevated INR with significant bleeding	
For less urgent situations	• Stop Coumadin and give slow IV vitamin K (10mg) • Supplement with 2 to 3 units fresh frozen plasma
For life-threatening situations	• Recombinant factor VIIa or Prothrombin complex concentrate (PCC)
* Identify and correct underlying factors for over anticoagulation like poor compliance, disease process, drugs etc.	

Table 7.7 Treatment of supratherapeutic INR from Coumadin toxicity

Warfarin toxicity can be reversed with various methods depending on the INR level. For patients with INR above therapeutic level, but still less than 5.0 can have a reduction in INR simply by withholding the dose for 24 hours and subsequently continue with a lower dose. Holding the dose of Coumadin usually lower the INR by 1 to 1.5 units per 24 hours. For INR levels above 5.0 can be treated with or without oral or intravenous vitamin K depending on whether the patient has active bleeding or not. Patients with high levels of INR associated with life-threatening bleeding complications should be treated with intravenous vitamin K and at times intravenous fresh frozen plasma to re-establish levels of clotting factors.

Antiplatelets

Aspirin

Aspirin is the oldest and most frequently used antiplatelet drug in modern medicine. Along with its antiplatelet properties, aspirin also acts as antipyretic, analgesic and anti-inflammatory agent. As an antiplatelet agent, Aspirin is used for *primary prevention of myocardial infarction* in patients with atherosclerotic heart disease. It is also used for *prevention of acute stroke* in patients with cerebrovascular disease and in selected patients with atrial fibrillation.

Aspirin produces its antiplatelet effect by *preventing the synthesis of prostaglandins.* Aspirin achieves this effect by *irreversibly inhibiting* **Cyclooxygenase 1 and 2** (**COX-1** and **COX-2**) enzymes that catalyze production of the prostaglandin derivative called **Thromboxane A_2**. Since ***Thromboxane A_2*** *is a potent platelet aggregator and vasoconstrictor*, *its inhibition results in antiplatelet effect*. Aspirin irreversibly affect Thromboxane A_2 and therefore the *platelets are inhibited from sticking together for the rest of their life span*.

Because of its antiplatelet function, Aspirin can cause bleeding complications especially in patients with coexisting conditions like gastrointestinal bleeding, use of warfarin or other antiplatelet or anticoagulant agents. In general, a lower doses of aspirin is well tolerated without any significant side-effects. **Aspirin allergy** manifested with *significant bronchospasm* is reported especially in patients with chronic urticaria, asthma, nasal polyps and chronic rhinitis. Overdose of Aspirin can cause hepatic and renal impairment since the drug is metabolized in liver and excreted through kidney.

Dipyridamole

Dipyridamole (**Persantine®**) is a *relatively weak antiplatelet agent* used in combination with low-dose aspirin (**Aggrenox®**) for prevention of stroke. Dipyridamole achieves its antiplatelet action by *blocking the breakdown of cyclic AMP* (**cAMP**). This process reduces platelet activation and cause vasodilation. Potent vasodilator effect of Dipyridamole is responsible for its major side effects like dizziness, flushing, headache and hypotension. Because of the availability of better antiplatelet medications without significant debilitating side effects (e.g. Clopidogrel), dipyridamole is not widely used as an antiplatelet agents anymore.

Thienopyridines

This group of antiplatelet agents exert their action by *selectively inhibiting* **P2Y12 component of ADP receptors** *on the* *platelet surface*. This in turn *prevent activation of* **glycoprotein IIb/IIIa receptor** complex and thereby platelet aggregation. **Thienopyridines** *irreversibly block these receptors* and therefore inhibitory effect remains active for the lifespan of the platelet (7 to 10 days). Major examples are **Ticlopidine** (**Ticlid®**), **Clopidogrel** (**Plavix®**) and **Prasugrel** (**Effient®**). Among these, Ticlopidine is falling out of favor because of the risk of life-threatening blood disorders like neutropenia, agranulocytosis and thrombotic thrombocytopenic purpura (TTP).

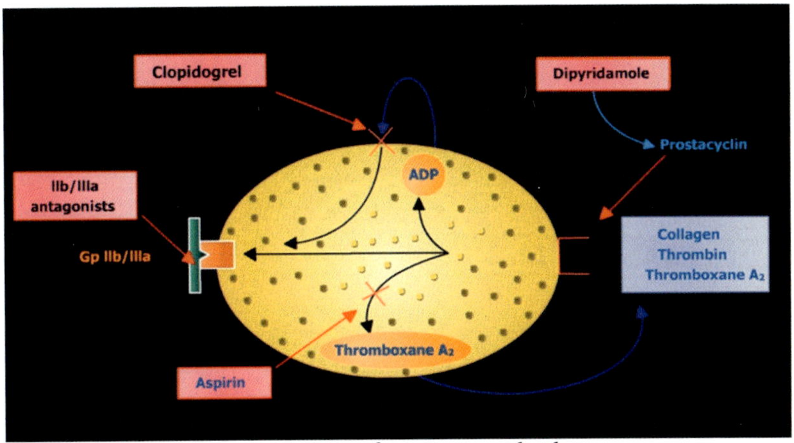

Fig 7.5 Action of various antiplatelets

Among these, Prasugrel has rapid onset of action than Clopidogrel and Ticlopidine. However, because of the increased risk of bleeding Prasugrel is reserved for selected patient population after percutaneous coronary intervention. Due to their irreversible nature of platelet inhibition, patients should be *off of Thienopyridines for an average of 5 to 7 days* before undergoing any major surgical intervention including Coronary Artery Bypass Grafting(CABG).

Cyclo Pentyl Triazolo Pyrimidines (**CPTP**)

This is a newer group of **P2Y12 ADP antagonist** with a *direct reversible inhibitory effect* on the platelets. These agents are more potent and have better clinical outcomes than that of Thienopyridines. They have similar side-effect profile with Thienopyridines. **Ticagrelor** (**Brilinta**), a reversible P2Y12 inhibitor is used as oral antiplatelet agent in patients with percutaneous coronary intervention and stent placement. Interestingly, *use of*

Aspirin with dosage more than 100 mg per day may reduce the efficacy of Ticagrelor.

Glycoprotein IIb/IIIa Receptor Antagonist (**IIb/IIIa Inhibitors**)

These are intravenous antiplatelet agents targeting the Glycoprotein receptors on the surface of the platelets. Even though IIb/IIIa receptors are most abundant receptors on the surface of the platelet, *they become active only when platelets are sensitized*. Upon activation, these receptors bind to the **Fibrinogen** and **von Willebrand Factor** (**vWF**) and cause platelet aggregation. These agents are particularly useful in patients undergoing coronary intervention for acute myocardial infarction with thrombus burden in the coronary arteries. Examples are **Abciximab** (**ReoPro®**),**Eptifibatide** (**Integrillin®**) and **Tirofiban** (**Aggrastat®**). Among these, **Eptifibatide** and **Tirofiban** *are synthetic molecules* with a short half-life whereas, **Abciximab** is a *fragment of an immunoglobulin* that targets glycoprotein IIb/IIIa receptors.

Factor Xa inhibitors

Oral factor Xa inhibitors, also known as **Noval Oral Anticoaguant** agents (NOAC) have rapid onset of action and predictable pharmacokinetics. Examples are **Dabigatran**(Pradaxa®), **Rivaroxaban** (Xarelto®) and **Apixaban** (Eliquis®), **Edoxaban** (Savaysa®), and **Betrixaban** (Bevyxxa®). Advantage of these agents in day-to-day use is their oral route of administration and lack of need for any close monitoring as in the case of Coumadin. Factor Xa Inhibitors are perfect for outpatient treatment of thromboembolic disorders like atrial fibrillation (non-valvular) and deep vein thrombosis (DVT).

New Anticoagulants under Development

Class of drug	Perceived benefit
Synthetic heparin pentasaccharide (An analogue of Fondaparinux) E.g. Idrabiotaparinux	Anti- factor Xa activity with weekly administration schedule
Ultra low molecule weight heparin	Pure Anti- factor Xa activity
Factor VIII inhibitor	Possibly one dose every 10 days
Recombinant human soluble Thrombomodulin (rhTM)	Possibly one dose every 5 to 6 days

Table 7.8 New anticoagulants under development

Drug	Onset/ peak	Half Life	Metabolism	Elimination
Heparin				
Unfractionated Heparin (UHF)	IV Immediate SubQ 20-30 min	Dose dependant (Average 1-2 hrs)	Hepatic	Urine
Low Molecular weight Heparin (LMWH)				
Enoxaparin *Lovenox®*	3-5 hrs(peak)	4.5-7 hrs	Hepatic	Urine
Dalteparin *Fragmin®*	1-2 hrs	2-5 hrs	Hepatic	Urine
Tinzaparin *Innohep®*	2-3 hrs	82 min	Hepatic	Urine
Synthetic low molecule weight heparin (Factor Xa Inhibitor)				
Fondaparinux *Arixtra®*	Rapid	17-21 hrs	Unknown	Urine
Direct Thrombin Inhibitors				
Lepirudin** *Refludan®*	Immediate	Less than 1 hr	Hepatic	Urine
Argatroban	Immediate	39-51 min	Hepatic	Feces and Urine
Bivalirudin *Angiomax®*	Immediate	25 min	Blood proteases	Urine
Desirudin *Iprivask®*	1-3 hrs (Subcutaneous)	2 hrs	Renal	Renal
Thrombolytics (Non Specific)				
Streptokinase** Streptase®	Immediate	23 min	None	Liver
Anistreplase Eminase®	Immediate	94 min	Plasma	None
Urokinase Kinlytic®	Immediate	20-30 min	Hepatic	Hepatic and renal
Thrombolytics (Specific)				
Alteplase Activase®	Immediate	35 min	Hepatic	Urine
Tenecteplase TNKase®	Immediate	90-130 min	Hepatic	Plasma
Reteplase Retavase®	Immediate	13-19 min	Liver	Feces and Urine

** Not available in USA

Table 7.9-A Pharmacokinetics of anticoagulants

Drug	Onset/ peak	Half Life	Metabolism	Elimination
Vitamin K antagonists				
Warfarin *Coumadin®*	24-72 hrs	20-60 hrs	Hepatic	Urine
Antiplatelets				
Aspirin	Immediate	Dose dependant 5-10 hrs	GI and Hepatic	Urine
Dipyridamole *Persantine®*	Immediate	10-12 hrs	Hepatic	Feces
Thienopyridines				
Ticlopidine *Ticlid®*	6 hrs	13 hrs	Hepatic	Urine and Feces
Clopidogrel *Plavix®*	Dose dependant 2-6 hr (loading dose)	6 hrs	Hepatic	Urine and Feces
Prasugrel *Effient®*	Dose dependant 30 min (loading dose)	2-15 hrs	Intestinal and Serum	Urine and Feces
Cyclopentyl Trlazolopyrimidines				
Ticagrelor *Brilinta®*	30 min (loading dose)	9 hrs	Hepatic	Feces and Urine
Glycoprotein IIb/IIIa receptor antagonist				
Abciximab *ReoPro®*	Rapid	30 min	None	Urine
Eptifibatide *Integrillin®*	<1 hr	2.5 hr	Minimal	Urine
Tirofiban *Aggrastat®*	Immediate	2 hrs	Minimal hepatic	Urine and Feces
Factor Xa inhibitors				
Dabigatran *Pradaxa®*	Immediate	12-17 hrs	Hepatic	Renal
Rivaroxaban *Xarelto®*	2-4 hr (peak)	11-13 hrs	Hepatic	Urine and Feces
Apixaban *Eliquis®*	3-4 hrs	Dose dependant 8-15 hrs	Hepatic	Urine and Feces
Endoxaban Savaysa®	1-2 hrs	10-14 hrs	Hepatic	Urine and Feces
Betrixaban Bevyxxa®	3-4 hrs	19-27 hrs	Minimal hepatic	Feces

Table 7.9-B Pharmacokinetics of anticoagulants

Points to remember!!!

- Major components of blood are **red blood cells** (Erythrocytes), **white blood cells** (Leukocytes) and **platelets** (Thrombocytes) suspended in **plasma**.
- **Erythrocytes** are *flexible biconcave disc shaped cells without a nucleus and contain* **hemoglobin**.
- Erythropoiesis is regulated by a substance called **Erythropoietin;** *released from the kidney.*
- White blood cells include **Granulocytes** (65%), **Lymphocytes** (30%) and **Monocytes** (5%). **Granulocytes** are further divided into **Neutrophils** (95%), **Eosinophils** (4%) and **Basophils** (1%).
- ***Granulocytes*** *and* ***Monocytes*** *are actively involved in defending the body against microbes* by attacking and engulfing foreign objects (**phagocytosis**)
- ***Lymphocytes*** *produce humoral and cell mediated immunity* through B-lymphocytes and T-lymphocytes.
- Platelets are the cell *fragments produced from disintegration of* **megakaryocytes**.
- The productions of platelets are regulated by a substance called **Thrombopoietin**.
- Platelets *provide both mechanical barrier and a platform for further coagulation process.*
- Platelets also contain and release **Serotonin** at the time of injury and *causes localized vasoconstriction.*
- Along with **Thromboxane A_2**, platelets also release **Prostacyclin I_2** (PGI_2) that *causes vasodilation and inhibition of platelet adherence*. Together they regulate platelet aggregation.
- The *bond between platelets and the injured vessel wall* (***platelet adherence***) is ensured by **von Willebrand factor** (**vWF**)
- **Calcium ions** also play a major role in platelet aggregation
- **Thromboxane A_2** facilitates activation of **glycoprotein IIb/**

IIIa receptors on the platelet surface, which in turn *exposes fibrinogen binding sites on the platelet surface.*

- **Coagulation cascade** is the pathway of blood coagulation and can be initiated by two different mechanisms called **extrinsic pathway** (**tissue pathway**) and **intrinsic pathway**.
- After a series of enzymatic activation, both of these pathways come down to a common series of chemical modulation known as **common pathway**.
- Fibrinolysis is the *enzymatic degradation of fibrin clot after the vessel injury is stabilized* and is carried out mainly by the enzyme called **Plasmin**.
- **Plasminogen** is the precursor of active plasmin and is synthesized in the liver.
- **Tissue plasminogen activator** (**t-PA**) and **Urokinase** *facilitate conversion of plasminogen to plasmin and thereby fibrinolysis.*
- The products of fibrin breakdown known as **fibrin degradation products** (**FDP**) themselves *act as potent anticoagulants.*
- *Unwanted coagulation process in the body is inhibited by a naturally occurring anticoagulation system* consists of **Antithrombin III**, **Heparin cofactor II**, **Protein C** and **Protein S**.
- Coagulation abnormalities are prevented by *maintaining a balance between the amount of activated clotting factors, inhibitors of coagulation and degradation of fibrin clot.*
- **Antithrombin III** is considered as a major inhibitor of coagulation and it slowly *inactivate active forms of clotting factors X, IX, XI, XII* and *thrombin.*
- **Heparin cofactor II** inhibits both **Thrombin** and **Thrombin induced platelet aggregation**. *Functions of both Antithrombin and heparin cofactor II are greatly increased in the presence of* **Heparin**.
- **Protein C** is a **vitamin K dependent protein**, synthesized in the liver and is circulated in the blood in its inactive form and get activated in to activated protein C by Thrombin.

- **Activated protein C (APC)** *inactivates* **Factor V$_a$** and **Factor VIII$_a$**.
- Protein C also promotes fibrinolysis by *inactivating inhibitors of t-PA* and thereby *facilitating conversion of plasminogen to plasmin.*
- **Protein S** acts as a cofactor for Protein C in *inactivation of* **factor V$_a$** and **factor VIII$_a$**.
- Unfractionated heparin acts as anticoagulants by augmenting *the inhibitory function of* **Antithrombin III** on clotting **factor II** (**Thrombin**), **XII**, **XI**, **IX** and **factor Xa**.
- Because of its *large structure, unfractionated heparin can attach to both* ***Thrombin*** *and* ***factor Xa***
- UFH has *immediate onset of action when given intravenously.*
- UFH has high *affinity for plasma proteins and other cellular components* in the blood and that *causes lower therapeutic benefits and increased chance of immunology reaction*
- UFH has a non-linear dose response approach in which a *small change in dosage can lead to large effect in anticoagulation response.*
- Adequacy of treatment with unfractionated heparin can be monitored by doing **activated Partial Thromboplastin Time** (**aPTT**).
- Heparin induced thrombocytopenia is usually seen in patients undergoing *prolonged treatment* (*>4 days*) using heparin.
- **Type I** (benign form) HIT is caused by **platelet sequestration**; usually happens in the beginning of the treatment, characterized by *platelet count rarely goes less than 100,000/mm^3 and resolves without any intervention and is clinically insignificant.*
- Type II HIT is **immune-mediated** with the *onset of symptoms from 5 to 15 days after heparin administration and also called* **White clot syndrome**.
- *Widespread platelet activation and subsequent aggregation* result in arterial and venous thrombosis secondary to the formation of antibodies against the **heparin-platelet factor 4**

complex (**PF4**).

- *Immediate discontinuation of all heparin sources* including heparin flushes is required until platelet count normalizes.

- Cross sensitivity between unfractionated and low molecule weight heparin prevents the use of LMWH during HIT.

- **Bivalirudin** (**Angiomax®**), **Argatroban** (both are *direct thrombin inhibitors*), **Fondaparinux** (**Arixtra®**- a *factor Xa inhibitor*) and **Lepirudin** (*recombinant Hirudin*) can be used during HIT.

- LMWH attains its *anticoagulation effect through* **antithrombin III** *activation and resulting* **factor Xa** *inhibition.*

- *LMWH has a better pharmacologic profile with a predictable action from patient to patient and a long half life.*

- **Antithrombin binding pentasaccharide** sequence called **Fondaparinux** only attaches to antithrombin III and get anticoagulation effect through factor Xa inhibition without affecting thrombin.

- **Direct thrombin inhibitors** *target* **thrombin** *molecule itself to achieve their anticoagulation effect.*

- The *most important clinical advantage of using direct thrombin inhibitors are their ability to inactivate the thrombin bound to the clot.*

- *Direct thrombin inhibitors do not interact with* **platelet factor (PF4)** which is responsible for **heparin induced thrombocytopenia**.

- *Argatroban is approved for treatment of HIT.*

- **Bivalirudin** (**Angiomax®**) is a *synthetic analogue of **Hirudin*** and is commonly *used for anticoagulation during* **percutaneous coronary intervention**.

- Fibrinolytics agents are performing their action through *conversion of* **plasminogen** *to active* **plasmin**.

- **First generation fibrinolytic agents** such as **Streptokinase**, **Anistreplace** and **Urokinase** are *non-specific for fibrin bound* *plasminogen* and therefore had more bleeding risk.

- Newer generation of **recombinant tissue plasminogen activator** (**rt-PA**) agents such as **Alteplase** or **Activase**, and its derivatives **Tenecteplase** (**TNKase®**) and **Reteplase** (**Retavase®**) are *fibrin bound plasminogen specific* and has a better clinical benefit.

- **Streptokinase** produces *hypotension* and has *immune-mediated effects that cause antibody production resulting in possible allergic reactions*.

- Coumadin achieves the anticoagulation effect through *inhibiting activation of* **vitamin K dependent** *clotting factors such as* **factor II**, **VII**, **IX** *and* **X and** *anticoagulants factors such as* **Protein C** and **Protein S**.

- Coumadin work through **extrinsic pathway** of clotting cascade and *interferes with the activation of inactive vitamin K into its active form*.

- Even though Coumadin affect the clotting factors, *it does not inactivate existing clotting factors* in the blood.

- Effectiveness of anticoagulation with Coumadin is monitored through **Prothrombin** and **International normalized ratio (INR)**.

- Patients at high risk for bleeding include *elderly clients, patients with congestive heart failure, underlying malignancy, severely impaired hepatic or renal dysfunction, inadequate nutrition, previous history of GI bleeding* etc.

- Common food items, especially **green leafy vegetables** affects therapeutic effect of Coumadin because of *their high vitamin K content*.

- Coumadin toxicity with high levels of INR associated with life-threatening bleeding complications should be treated with **intravenous vitamin K** and at times **intravenous fresh frozen plasma**

- Aspirin is an antiplatelet agent used for *primary prevention of myocardial infarction* and *prevention of acute stroke*.

- Aspirin produces its antiplatelet effect by *preventing the synthesis of prostaglandins by irreversibly inhibiting*

Cyclooxygenase 1 and 2 and **Thromboxane A_2**.

- ***Thromboxane A_2*** *is a potent platelet aggregator and vasoconstrictor* and *it's inhibition results in antiplatelet effect.*

- Dipyridamole (**Persantine®**) is a *relatively weak antiplatelet agent* used in combination with low-dose aspirin (**Aggrenox®**) for prevention of stroke.

- **Thienopyridines** antiplatelet agents exert their action by *selectively inhibiting* **P2Y12 component of ADP receptors** *on the platelet surface*

- Patients should be *off of Thienopyridines for an average of 5 to 7 days* before undergoing any major surgical intervention.

- Cyclopentyl Triazolopyrimidines is a class of **P2Y12 ADP antagonist** with *direct reversible inhibitory effect* on the platelets. E.g. **Ticagrelor**

- *Use of Aspirin with dosage more than 100 mg per day may reduce the efficacy* of Ticagrelor

- **Glycoprotein IIb/IIIa receptor antagonist** (**IIb/IIIa inhibitors**) are intravenous antiplatelet agents targeted at the Glycoprotein receptors on the surface of the platelets**. E**xamples are **Abciximab** (**ReoPro®**),**Eptifibatide** (**Integrillin®**) and **Tirofiban** (**Aggrastat®**).

- **Oral factor Xa inhibitors** like **Dabigatran**(Pradaxa®), **Rivaroxaban** (Xarelto®) and **Apixaban** (Eliquis®), **Endoxaban** (Savaysa®), and **Betrixaban** (Bevyxxa®) have rapid onset of action and predictable pharmacokinetics and does not need for any close monitoring .

8 Nitrates and Vasodilators

Vasodilators in general can be classified into venous vasodilators, arterial vasodilators and balanced vasodilators. Among them, **venous vasodilators** *cause peripheral venous dilation leading to a reduction in venous blood flow* coming back to the heart. They are also known as preload reductors. **Arterial vasodilators** impart *relaxation of arteries* and thereby *reduction in the pressure against which the heart has to pump*, known as afterload reductors. Some agents cause *both arterial and venous vasodilatation in a balanced fashion*, called **balanced vasodilators**.

Nitrates

Nitroglycerin

Nitrates are the mainstay agents in treatment of angina in patients with coronary artery disease. Used as an explosive compound in the beginning dates of its discovery, nitrates are one of the *oldest and actively used drugs* over last 130 years. Nitrates impart their pharmacologic action by *relaxing vascular smooth muscles*. Relaxation of venous circulatory system results in *reduction of preload and thereby myocardial oxygen demand*. In higher doses, they can impart significant arterial dilation as well.

They also have *preferential relaxation effect on the coronary vasculature*, resulting in redistribution of blood flow from normally perfused to ischemic areas of the myocardium. This redistribution effect is believed to be because of their action on improving collateral circulation and also reducing ventricular diastolic pressure, which in turn reduce subendocardial compression. This effect has been successfully demonstrated in patients with chronic angina, where nitroglycerin increases blood flow by redistribution without affecting global myocardial perfusion. They also *prevent vasoconstriction caused by* endothelial dysfunction in areas of myocardium deprived of adequate circulation. Even though clinically not significant, nitroglycerin also acts as an **antithrombotic agent** by inhibiting platelet aggregation and facilitating vasodilatation.

Mechanism of action of nitroglycerin is through its conversion into **active nitric oxide** (**NO**), which subsequently activates production of intracellular **cyclic Guanosine Monophosphate** (**cGMP**). This product is *responsible for vasodilator and antiplatelet effect of nitroglycerin*. Until recently (till 2002), the exact biochemical mechanism behind nitrate's function was unknown. Now we know that **Mitochondrial aldehyde dehydrogenase** is *the enzyme responsible for biotransformation of nitrates* in the body. It is also believed to be the enzyme responsible for **nitrate tolerance** that is described later in this chapter. Some of the experiments have shown that *long-term use of nitroglycerin preparations can impair the endothelial relaxation effect of nitroglycerin* by generation of free radicals.

Nitroglycerin is available in sublingual tablets, sublingual spray, tropical ointment, transdermal patches and intravenous preparation. Because of the *extensive hepatic first pass metabolism*, *oral preparations of nitroglycerin are not generally used as immediate acting agents* for relief of angina.

Nitroglycerin Preparations

Sublingual preparations of nitroglycerin are available in both tablet and metered dose spray forms. Since *sublingual administration bypasses first pass metabolism*, *a transient therapeutic dose of nitroglycerin is available* in the circulatory system for immediate effect. The usual dose is 0.3 to 0.6 mg with a maximum dose of 1.2 mg/15 min. Patients are instructed to take one sublingual tablet or spray in every 5 min up to 3 doses for symptom relief.

Nitroglycerin has a relatively short half-life (**1 to 3 min**) and then it will be converted to inactive metabolites. *Complete clinical effect of nitroglycerin is reversed within 30 to 60 min* because of hepatic metabolism. These agents can also be used for angina prophylaxis by using them 5 to 10 min before physical activity.

There are two forms of oral preparations available known as **Isosorbide dinitrate** and **Isosorbide 5-mononitrate**. Among them, **Isosorbide dinitrate** *has extensive first pass metabolism in the liver* *resulting in low bioavailability*. It is available as sublingual or as sustained release tablet form for oral administration. **Isosorbide mononitrate** *is an active metabolite of Isosorbide dinitrate and is completely bioavailable* because of its lack of first pass hepatic metabolism. It has a half-life of 4 to 6 hours and therefore can be used for treatment of **chronic stable angina**. Isosorbide mononitrate is available as sustained release preparation (continuous low-dose release of active nitroglycerin).

Topical preparations of nitroglycerin include ointment and transdermal patches. With duration of action of 4 to 6 hours, nitroglycerin ointment is applied on the chest wall for patients with angina pectoris. The *skin permeability of the drug is increased with hydration*. In transdermal patches, the drug reservoir is shielded from the skin with a semi permeable membrane that allows a sustained low-dose release (usually 0.1 -0.8 mg/hr).

Intravenous form of nitroglycerin is used only in critical care setting under close monitoring. This is commonly used for *treatment of angina in patients with acute myocardial infarction and also for management of hypertension* through peripheral vasodilation. It has beneficial effect in patients with *congestive heart failure and hypertension* because of its preload reducing effect.

Adverse Reactions

Common adverse reactions of nitroglycerin are related to its relaxation effect on vascular structures. *Headache*, *flushing* and *hypotension* are the most common adverse reactions. Among these, hypotension can be serious in patients with volume depletion and low vascular reserve like elderly and seriously ill. In these patients, *changing posture to upright from lying position can initiate symptomatic bradycardia and vasovagal syncope*.

> Instruct the patients to avoid use of any forms of nitroglycerin including sublingual tablets while taking **Phosphodiesterace-5 (PDE-5) inhibitors** such as **Sildenafil** (**Viagra®**) **Tadalafil** (**Cialis®**) etc, which are commonly used for treatment of organic erectile dysfunction. Concomitant use can cause profound and potentially life-threatening hypotensive episodes. These patients are to avoid taking either nitroglycerin or PDE-5 within 24 to 36 hours of one another.

Nitrates tolerance is another complication that can happen with prolonged use of this drug. **Tolerance** is defined as the *inability of the vascular epithelium to respond with vasodilation after sustained use of the drug*. This can be avoided by having nitrate free intervals during treatment. When using transdermal preparations of nitroglycerin, the patients are advised to take the patch off after 12 hours in a 24 hour window, thereby creating a nitrate free interval to prevent tolerance. Nitrate withdrawal in the form of worsening of angina after discontinuation of long-acting nitrates is also demonstrated. It can be prevented by co-administration of other anti-anginal agents like beta-blockers or calcium channel blockers.

Sodium Nitroprusside **(Nipride/Nitropress)**

It is a *potent fast-acting arterial and venous vasodilator* (balanced vasodilator) that performs its function through the active metabolite of Nitric oxide (**NO**). Because of its *very short half-life, Nitroprusside is given as continuous IV infusion*. It has rapid onset and offset of action that facilitate fine titration of the dose in clinical situations like **hypertensive crisis**, **acute decompensated heart failure** and **acute mitral regurgitation**. Because of its extreme potency and possibility of causing severe hypotension, *continuous hemodynamic monitoring through an arterial line is essential* for adequate titration. In patients with coronary artery disease,

> In patients with severe coronary artery disease, administration of rapid acting vasodilators such as Nitroprusside can cause diversion of blood supply from narrowed arteries leading to ischemia called coronary steal syndrome. In patients with coronary artery disease, arteries in the areas without narrowing are maintained at higher resistance in order to maintain adequate flow into the parts of the heart with arterial narrowing. Generalized vasodilation of these patent vessels practically lowers the amount of blood going into the ischemic areas. Because of the same reason, Sodium Nitroprusside may not be an ideal agent for treatment of hypertensive crisis in patients with myocardial infarction.

generalized vasodilatation can cause coronary steal syndrome as described in the box.

Sodium Nitroprusside can also cause hypoxemia in patients with COPD because of ventilation-perfusion mismatch in the pulmonary circulation. Another major adverse reaction from prolonged use of Nitroprusside is **cyanide toxicity**. *Patients with renal dysfunction are at high risk of having this complication*. Therefore, Sodium Nitroprusside is used only for short duration. During treatment, these patients should be monitored for *signs of cyanide toxicity like nausea, vomiting and central nervous system disturbances*. If suspected, infusion should be stopped immediately and **3% Sodium Nitrite** should be given.

Nesiritide (Natrecor)

It is a *recombinant form of* **human Brain Natriuretic Peptide** (**BNP**) that causes **balanced vasodilation** leading to *increase in cardiac output independent of ionotropic or chronotropic aspects* of the heart. It has *longer half-life than that of Nitroglycerin and*

Drug	Onset/ peak	Half Life	Metabolism	Elimination
Nitroglycerin (Venous vasodilators)				
Sublingual Tab /spray *Nitrolingual®*	1-3 min	1-4 min	Hepatic	Urine
Topical ointment *Nitro-Bid®*	10-30 min	1-4 min	Hepatic	Urine
Transdermal patch *Nitro-Dur®*	30 min	1-4 min	Hepatic	Urine
Extended release *Imdur®*	30-60 min	5-6 hrs	Hepatic	Urine
Extended release *Isordil®*	1 hr	5 hrs	Extensive hepatic	Urine and Feces
Balance Vasodilators				
Sodium Nitroprusside *Nipride®, Nitropress®*	<2 min	2 min	Erythrocytes Liver	Urine
Nesiritide *Natrecor®*	15 min	18 min	Vascular system	Urine
Direct Arterial Vasodilators				
Hydralazine *Apresoline®*	Oral 20-30 min IV 5-20 min	2-8 hrs 7-16 hrs in renal dysfunction	Extensive first pass	Urine
Minoxidil *Loniten®*	<30 min	3.5-4.2 hrs	Liver	Urine

Table 8.1 Pharmacokinetics of vasodilators

Sodium Nitroprusside. It is also used for treatment of acutely decompensated congestive heart failure. Like Nitroglycerin, Nesiritide also exerts its pharmacologic action through *stimulation of* **cyclic GMP** that facilitates vascular smooth muscle relaxation. This drug also has *a short half-life of 18 min* and therefore should be given as a continuous infusion.

Direct Arterial Vasodilators

Hydralazine (**Apresoline®**) and **Minoxidil** (**Loniten®**) cause *predominant arterial vasodilation with a little or no effect on the venous system*. Therefore, these agents act as **afterload reductors**. They are particularly useful in *treatment of severe hypertension*. Among these, Minoxidil is more potent and is useful for severe refractory hypertension in patients with renal insufficiency. **Minoxidil** attains its *therapeutic effect by opening potassium channels* in the vascular smooth muscle.

Because of the property of fluid retention and possibility of *reflex tachycardia from sympathetic response*, *these agents should be used along with a diuretic and a beta-blocker* to avoid side effects. Because of its ability to increase cutaneous blood flow and stimulation of resting hair follicles, **Minoxidil** *can cause excessive hair growth* and can be a problem especially in women. Because of the same property, Minoxidil in topical formulation is used for treatment of alopecia.

Points to remember!!!

- Vasodilators in general can be classified into **venous vasodilators**, **arterial vasodilators** and **balanced vasodilators**.
- **Venous vasodilators** *cause peripheral venous dilation leading to a reduction in venous flow* coming back to the heart. They are also known as **preload reductors**.
- **Arterial vasodilators** impart *relaxation of arteries and thereby reduction in the pressure against which the heart has to pump*; known as **afterload reductors**.
- Some agents cause *both arterial and venous vasodilatation in a balanced fashion*, called **balanced vasodilators**.
- Nitrates impart their pharmacologic action by *relaxing vascular*

smooth muscles.

- Relaxation of venous circulatory system results in *reduction of preload and thereby myocardial oxygen demand.*
- They also have *preferential relaxation effect on the coronary vasculature* resulting in redistribution of blood flow from normally perfused to ischemic areas of the myocardium.
- They also *prevent vasoconstriction caused by* **endothelial dysfunction** in areas of myocardium deprived of adequate circulation.
- Nitroglycerin also acts as an **antithrombotic agent** by inhibiting platelet aggregation and facilitating vasodilatation.
- Mechanism of action of nitroglycerin is through its conversion into **active nitric oxide** (**NO**), which subsequently activates production of intracellular **cyclic Guanosine Monophosphate** (**cGMP**). This product is *responsible for vasodilator and antiplatelet effect of nitroglycerin.*
- *Long-term use of nitroglycerin preparations can impair the endothelial relaxation effect of nitroglycerin* by generation of free radicals.
- Because of their *extensive hepatic first pass metabolism, oral preparations of fast-acting nitroglycerin are not generally used as immediate acting agents* for relief of angina.
- *Complete clinical effect of nitroglycerin is reversed within 30 to 60 min* because of hepatic metabolism.
- **Isosorbide dinitrate** *has extensive first pass metabolism in the liver resulting in low bioavailability.*
- **Isosorbide mononitrate** *is an active metabolite of Isosorbide dinitrate and is completely bioavailable.* It has longer half life and can be used for treatment of chronic stable angina.
- *Headache, flushing* and *hypotension* are the most common adverse reactions from Nitroglycerine.
- **Nitrates tolerance** is a complication that can happen with prolonged use and is defined as the *inability of the vascular*

epithelium to respond with vasodilation after sustained use of the drug.

- **Nitrates tolerance** can be avoided by having **nitrate free intervals** during treatment.
- **Sodium Nitroprusside** is a *potent fast-acting arterial and venous vasodilator* (**balanced vasodilator**).
- Because of its *very short half-life, Nitroprusside is given as continuous IV infusion in situations like* hypertensive crisis, acute decompensated heart failure and acute mitral regurgitation.
- In patients with coronary artery disease, generalized vasodilatation can cause **coronary steal syndrome**
- Sodium Nitroprusside can also cause hypoxemia in patients with COPD because of **ventilation-perfusion mismatch**
- Prolonged use of Nitroprusside can cause **cyanide toxicity** especially in patients with underlying renal dysfunction.
- *Signs of cyanide toxicity are nausea, vomiting and central nervous system disturbances*. If suspected, infusion should be stopped immediately and **3% Sodium Nitrite** should be given.
- **Nesiritide (Natrecor)** is a *recombinant form of* **human Brain Natriuretic Peptide** (**BNP**) that causes **balanced vasodilation**
- **Nesiritide** has *longer half-life than that of Nitroglycerin and Sodium Nitroprusside; however, still relatively short and therefore can only be given in continuous infusion.*
- **Hydralazine** (**Apresoline®**) and **Minoxidil** (**Loniten®**) cause *predominant arterial vasodilation with a little or no effect on the venous system (afterload reductors).*
- Because of the property of fluid retention and possibility of *reflex tachycardia from sympathetic response, direct arterial vasodilators should be used along with a diuretic and a beta-blocker*
- **Minoxidil** *can cause excessive hair growth* and can be a problem especially in women.

9 Inotropes and Vasopressors

These are the most common intravenous medications used in management of critical illnesses in intensive care unit. There are two types of agents commonly used in practice known as Vasopressors and Inotropes. Even though they fundamentally differ in their action, many of the drugs have both vasopressor and ionotropic properties.

Ionotropic agents increase intracellular cyclic Adenosine Monophosphate (**cAMP**) and thereby increasing intracellular calcium ions. Desired pharmacologic action of Inotropes are achieved through *stimulation of various adrenergic receptors* such as alpha-1, beta-1, beta-2 and dopamine receptors or *by preventing degradation of cAMP by inhibition of enzyme* Phosphodiesterase III (PDE-III).

Receptor Physiology	
Alpha-1 receptors	• Located in arterioles • Mediate **vasoconstriction**
Alpha-2 receptors	• They **inhibit Norepinephrine release** from sympathetic nerve endings
Beta-1 receptors	• Common in the atria, ventricles and AV node • Cause increasing contractility (**ionotropic effect**) and increase in heart rate (**chronotropic effect**).
Beta-2 receptors	• They are seen in arteries, arterioles, veins and bronchioles. • Stimulation results in **peripheral vasodilation**
Dopamine receptors	• They are located in the renal, mesenteric, coronary and cerebral vasculature. • Stimulation can cause **vasodilation**.

Table 9.1 Receptor physiology

Vasopressors on the other hand, influence peripheral vasculature and cause *vasoconstriction,* resulting in *increased mean arterial pressure* (MAP). Vasopressors are commonly indicated in clinical situations with a drop of > 30 mmHg systolic blood pressure from the baseline or mean arterial pressure (MAP) <60 mmHg.

Drug	Alpha-1	Alpha-2	Beta -1	Beta-2	Dopaminergic
Phenylephrine	+++				
Norepinephrine	+++	+++	++		
Epinephrine					
Low dose			++	+++	
Moderate dose	+		+++	+++	
High dose	+++	+++	+++	+++	
Dobutamine	+		+++	++	
Isoproterenol			+++	+++	
Dopamine (mcg/Kg/min)					
0.5-2			+		++
5-10	+		++		++
10-20	++		++		++

+ Weak effect; ++ Moderate effect; +++ Strong effect

Table 9.2 Receptor stimulation of Sympathomimetic agents

Clinical Effect of Sympathomimetic Agents

Drug	Receptor activity	Inotropic effect	Chronotropic effect	Vascular effect	Clinical effect
Isoproterenol	β1 > β2	+++	+++	Vasodilation	CO↑, SVR↓
Epinephrine (Dose dependant)	β1 = β2 > α	++	++	Vasoconstriction	CO↑↑ SVR↓ (Low dose) SVR↑ (High Dose)
Norepinephrine	α > β1 >β2	+	+	Vasoconstriction	SVR↑↑, CO ↔
Dopamine	β , α, dopamine	++	+	Vasoconstriction	CO↑ SVR↑ (Mod dose) SVR↑↑(High dose)
Dobutamine	β1 > β2 > α	++	+	Vasodilation	CO↑,SVR↓
Phenylephrine	α			Strong vasoconstriction	SVR↑↑, CO ↔

+++ Strong effect ; ++ Moderate effect; + Weak effect; ↑- Increase; ↑↑- Strongly increase; ↓- Decrease; ↔ No significant changes; CO- Cardiac Output; SVR- Systemic Vascular Resistance

Table 9.3 Clinical effects of sympathomimetic agents

Practical Points While Administering Sympathomimetic Agents

Drug Selection: Select the initial agent based on underlying etiology (e.g. Norepinephrine in cardiac failure with significant hypotension) and titrate for response. Add second agent if needed to compliment the effect.

Route of administration: Always use a central venous access if available to avoid risk of peripheral extravasation and subsequent tissue necrosis.

Tachyphylaxis: Important to remember that with long term use, sympathomimetic agents can cause tachyphylaxis where receptors are no longer able to respond adequately as before with simple dose increase.

Volume replacement: In order for Vasopressors to work, there should be adequate circulatory fluid volume and is especially important while treating septic shock.

Inadequate absorption of drugs: While on Vasopressors, drugs that are subcutaneously administered such as Insulin or heparin can have poor absorption due to cutaneous vasoconstriction.

Box 9.1 Practical points for sympathomimetic drugs

These conditions can result in hypo perfusion and end organ damage. Ionotropic and Vasopressor agents are commonly used in various types of shock, anaphylaxis, severe congestive heart failure etc.

Phenylephrine (**Neo-Synephrine®**)

It is a *synthetic catecholamine with selective* **alpha-1 agonist** function, resulting in **peripheral vasoconstriction** with minimal effect on heart rate and contractility. Phenylephrine is particularly useful in clinical situations with hypotension from systemic vasodilation and preserved cardiac output such as **septic shock**, **neurologic disorders** or **anesthesia induced hypotension**. Less potent preparations are used as nasal decongestents. Because of its potent vasoconstrictive effects, Phenylephrine can affect *absorption of subcutaneously administered drugs like insulin and heparin*.

Isoproterenol (Isuprel®)

This is a prominent **beta-1 receptor stimulant** with very minimal beta-2 receptor activity. This beta-2 receptor activity is more seen in higher doses. Strong beta-1 selective receptor activity of Isoproterenol leads to **positive ionotropic** (increasing contractility) and **positive chronotropic** (increase in heart rate) effect on the heart. It is commonly used for assessing **Neuro-cardiogenic syncope** while doing tilt table test and also during electrophysiologic assessments to induce arrhythmias.

Because of the strong beta agonist effect of isoproterenol, it can also be used as treatment of **beta-blocker overdose**. Even though not FDA approved, Isoproterenol is used in applications like *inducing override pacing for refractory torsade de pointes*, *control bradycardia in denervated heart transplant patients refractory to atropine*, *ventricular arrhythmias due to AV nodal blocking*, *electrical storm associated with Brugada syndrome* etc. It has immediate onset of action with a half-life of 2.5 to 5 min with intravenous administration.

> Extravasation of many Vasopressors and Inotropes in to the local tissue can cause tissue necrosis and therefore these agents are ideally infused through central venous catheter. **Phentolamine**, a strong alpha antagonist is used for treatment of extravasation from these agents.

Epinephrine (Adrenalin®)

Epinephrine is a very potent **Alpha and Beta receptor agonist** that can produce strong inotropic and chronotropic responses in the heart along with peripheral vasoconstriction. In all accounts, epinephrine is a **true sympathetic stimulant** and therefore highly used in treatment of cardiac arrest. Epinephrine is also used for treatment of anaphylactic reactions. As part of the adrenergic stimulation, epinephrine may increase ectopic pacemaker activity in the heart leading to arrhythmia. Epinephrine has some dose dependant responses. In lower to moderate doses, it has very minimal alpha receptor action. Epinephrine is available in multiple dosing combinations. Specifics of dosing and indications are explained in the table.

Use and Dosage of Epinephrine		
Indication	**Route**	**Dose**
Asystole/ PEA	IV or IO	1 mg Q 3-5 min
	Endotracheal	2-2.5 Q 3-5 min
Symptomatic bradycardia unresponsive to pacing or Atropine	IV infusion	2-10 mcg/min or 0.1- 0.5 mcg/Kg/min
Anaphylaxis	IM or SubQ (1:1000 or 1mg/mL)	0.2-0.5 mg Q 5-15 min
	IV (1:10,000 or 0.1mg/mL)	0.1mg over 5 min 5-15 mcg/min if profoundly hypotensive
	Self administration	0.3 mg May repeat 5-15 min if symptoms persist
Severe Hypotension and shock**	IV infusion	0.1-0.5 mcg/Kg/min
Bronchodilator	SubQ (1:1000 or 1mg/mL)	0.3-0.5 mg Q 20 min for 3 doses

** Unlabelled use

Table 9.4 Uses and dosage of Epinephrine

Norepinephrine **(Levophed®)**

Norepinephrine is a catecholamine with **strong Alpha receptor stimulating effect** than Beta receptors. It is commonly used to increase systemic vascular resistance. This increase in systemic vascular resistance essentially improves coronary circulation in severe hypotension. Because of its *less potent ionotropic and chronotropic activity*, *theoretically it is a better agent than Dopamine or Dobutamine in cardiogenic shock*. It is also used for treatment of septic shock. Norepinephrine should be used continuously because of rapid onset of action and short half-life of 1 to 2 min.

Milrinone **(Primacor®)**

It is a **Phosphodiesterase-3** (**PDE-3**) **inhibitor** used for short-term circulatory support in patients with advanced heart failure.Milrinone has a selective Phosphodiesterase inhibitor activity through which it maintain higher level of **cAMP** in cardiac and vascular tissues. This leads to **vasodilation** and **ionotropic effect**. Milrinone has *very little chronotropic stimulation*. Milrinone should be used with extreme caution in patients with coronary artery disease because of the incidence of long-term mortality from atrial and ventricular arrhythmias.

Dopamine

Dopamine is a member of organic catecholamine family with significant dose-dependent cardiovascular effects. Endogenous dopamine also acts as a **neurotransmitter** in the brain through dopamine receptors. Interestingly, *the intravenous drug Dopamine cannot cross the blood brain barrier* and therefore doesn't have any central nervous system effects. Dopamine produces dose-dependent actions ranging from coronary, renal and mesenteric vasodilation at lower doses to significant ionotropic, chronotropic and vasoconstrictive effects at higher doses. Dose-dependent response of dopamine is shown in the box.

Dose-dependent Response of Dopamine

Dose	Clinical response
≤2 mcg/Kg/min	Increase renal, coronary and mesenteric blood flow (**Vasodilator effect**).
5 to10 mcg/Kg/min	Causes **positive ionotropic** and **chronotropic** effect through beta-1 adrenergic receptor activation. (**Adrenergic effect**)
10-20 mcg/Kg/min	Causes alpha-1 receptor activation leading to **vasoconstriction** and **increase in systemic vascular resistance** (Vasoconstrictive or 'pressor' effect)

Table 9.5 Dose-dependent response of Dopamine

Dobutamine

Dobutamine is a sympathomimetic drugs that stimulates both **beta-1** and **beta-2 receptors** with little or no effect on Alpha receptors. Therefore, Dobutamine **increases cardiac output** and **heart rate** however, does not increase peripheral vascular resistance. Compared to Dopamine, *Dobutamine does not cause high incidence of tachycardia and ventricular arrhythmia*. In post myocardial infarction and congestive heart failure patients, Dobutamine is preferred over Dopamine because of the less incidence of tachycardia as well as afterload reduction from peripheral vasodilation (beta-2 effect).

Usual dose of administration of Dobutamine ranges from 2 to 20 mcg/kg/min. At *lower doses*, *Dobutamine performs as a pure nonselective beta adrenergic agent*. At higher doses it starts showing Alpha receptor function in the form of peripheral vasoconstriction. Dobutamine can reduce renal blood flow and therefore in some cases low-dose dopamine (1 to 2mcg/kg/min) is used along with Dobutamine to ensure adequate renal perfusion. Dopamine and

Indication	Dosage	Onset	Half Life	Contraindication	Side effects
Phenylephrine (Neo-Synephrine®)					
Hypotension/Shock	**IV bolus** 100-500mcg Q 10-15 min **IV infusion** 0.5mcg/Kg/min	**IM/SQ** 10-15 min **IV** Immediate	2-3 hrs	• Hypersensitivity • Severe hypertension • Ventricular tachycardia	Do not use within 14 days of MAOI therapy (cause severe hypertension)
Refractory Paroxysmal SVT	**IV bolus** 250-500 mcg over 30 sec				
Isoproterenol (Isuprel®)					
Brady arrhythmia, AV nodal block, Refractory Torsades de Pointes	**IV infusion** 2-10 mcg/min	Immediate	2.5 to 5 min	• Angina • ventricular arrhythmias • tachyarrhythmia	increase myocardial oxygen demand
Brugada syndrome with electrical storm**	**IV bolus** 1-2 mcg **Infusion** 0.15-0.3 mcg/min for 1 day				
Tilt table testing	**IV infusion** 1mcg/min (max 5 mcg/min)				
Norepinephrine (Levophed®)					
Hypotension/shock	**IV infusion** 8-12 mcg/min; **maintenance** 2 to 4 mcg/min	rapid	1 min	• Hypersensitivity • Hypovolemia	Long-term use with high dose causes severe peripheral vasoconstriction
Milrinone (Primacor®)					
CHF, Cardiac output maintenance	50 mcg/Kg IV over 10 min; then 0.375-0.75 mcg/Kg/min infusion	5 to 15 min	2.5 hours	hypersensitivity	Atrial or ventricular arrhythmias Hepatotoxicity Hypotension
Dopamine					
Hemodynamic support	1-20 mcg/Kg/min	5 min	2 min	Ventricular fibrillation pheochromocytoma	Tachyarrhythmia tissue necrosis if infiltrated
Dobutamine					
Cardiac decompensation	2-20 mcg/Kg/min	1 to 10 min	2 min	Hypersensitivity Idiopathic hypertrophic subaortic stenosis (IHSS)	Ventricular ectopy, Tachycardia

** Unlabelled use

Table 9.6 Major Inotrops and Vasopressors

Dobutamine should be used with extreme caution in patients with atrial or ventricular arrhythmias, pheochromocytoma, hypertrophic obstructive cardiomyopathy, severe aortic stenosis etc.

Points to remember!!!

- **Ionotropic agents** increase intracellular **cyclic Adenosine Monophosphate** (**cAMP**) and thereby increasing **intracellular calcium** ions.

- Pharmacologic action of Inotropes are achieved through *stimulation of various adrenergic receptors* such as **alpha-1**, **beta-1**, **beta-2** and **dopamine receptors** or *by preventing degradation of cAMP by inhibition of enzyme* **Phosphodiesterase III** (PDE-III).

- **Vasopressors** influence peripheral vasculature and cause *vasoconstriction* results in *increase in mean arterial pressure* (MAP).

- **Phenylephrine** (**Neo-Synephrine®**) is a *synthetic catecholamine with selective* **alpha-1 agonist** function; resulting in **peripheral vasoconstriction** with minimal effect on heart rate and contractility.

- Phenylephrine is particularly useful in clinical situations with hypotension from systemic vasodilation and preserved cardiac output such as **septic shock**, **neurologic disorders** or **anesthesia induced hypotension**.

- Because of its potent vasoconstrictive effects, Phenylephrine can affect *absorption of drugs such as insulin and heparin that are administered subcutaneously*.

- **Isoproterenol (Isuprel®)** is a prominent **beta-1 receptor stimulant** with very minimal beta-2 receptor activity causing **positive ionotropic** (increasing contractility) and **positive chronotropic** (increase in heart rate) effect on the heart.

- Because of the strong beta agonists' effect of isoproterenol, it can also be used as treatment of **beta-blocker overdose**.

- Epinephrine is a very potent **Alpha and Beta receptor agonist** with strong inotropic and chronotropic properties in the heart along with peripheral vasoconstriction (true sympathetic stimulant).

- Norepinephrine is a catecholamine with **strong Alpha receptor stimulating effect** and is commonly used to increase systemic vascular resistance. This increase in systemic vascular resistance essentially improves coronary circulation in severe hypotension.
- Norepinephrine should be used continuously because of rapid onset of action and short half-life of 1 to 2 min.
- **Milrinone (Primacor®)** is a Phosphodiesterase-3 (PDE-3) inhibitor used for short-term circulatory support in patients with advanced heart failure; causing **vasodilation** and **ionotropic effect** with very minimal chronotropic stimulation.
- Milrinone should be used with extreme caution in patients with coronary artery disease because of the incidence of long-term mortality from atrial and ventricular arrhythmias.
- Dopamine is a member of organic catecholamine family with significant dose-dependent cardiovascular renal and mesenteric effects.
- Dobutamine is a sympathomimetic drugs that stimulates both **beta-1** and **beta-2 receptors** with little or no effect on Alpha receptors.
- Dobutamine **increases cardiac output** and **heart rate**; however, does not increase peripheral vascular resistance.
- Compared to Dopamine, *Dobutamine does not cause high incidence of tachycardia and ventricular arrhythmia*.
- At *lower doses, Dobutamine performs as a pure nonselective beta adrenergic agent* and in higher doses, it starts showing Alpha receptor function in the form of peripheral vasoconstriction.
- Dobutamine can reduce renal blood flow and therefore in some cases low-dose dopamine (1 to 2mcg/kg/min) is used along with Dobutamine to ensure adequate renal perfusion.

10 Lipid Lowering Agents

In the last few decades, lipid lowering drugs received unusual attention from scholars around the world because of the knowledge regarding the role of lipid metabolism in development of atherosclerotic cardiovascular disease. Coronary artery disease, being one of the major causes of death in United States, tackling this pathophysiologic process becomes a huge priority for everyone involved. This leads to extensive investigation about the biochemical processes behind lipid metabolism and development of a number of drugs to prevent troubling consequences. In nutshell, lipid management is the core of preventive cardiovascular medicine. In order to better understand the mechanism of various lipid lowering drugs and their clinical effect, it is important to establish a solid foundation on the relation between lipid metabolism and atherosclerosis.

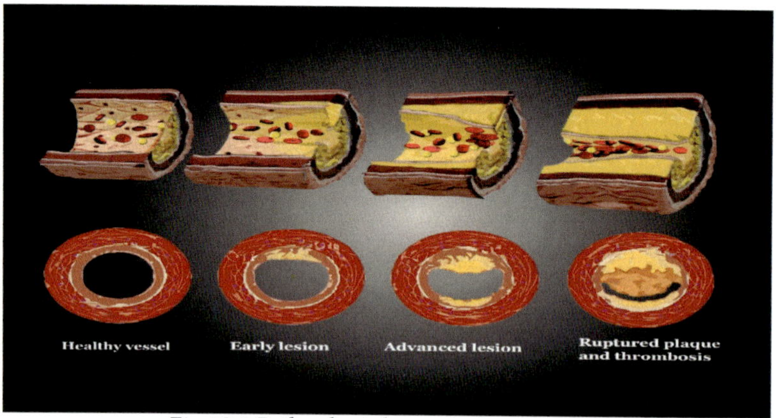

Fig 10.1 Pathophysiology of atherosclerosis

Lipoproteins

Major plasma lipids are **Cholesterol**, **Cholesteryl esterase**, **Triglycerides** and **Phospholipids**. Cholesterol is an *essential component of cell membranes that helps in steroid* *hormone production and bile acid formation*. Majority of circulating cholesterol is **Cholesteryl esterase** that forms the core of the lipoproteins. **Triglycerides** serve as a major form of stored energy and **Phospholipids** aid in lipid transportation and cellular function. Since the lipid molecules are insoluble in plasma, they are surrounded by transport molecules called **lipoproteins**. In this complex structure, the protein component is called **apolipoprotein** or apoproteins (**apo**). These are specialized proteins that identify specific receptors to which the lipid particles interact. Therefore, the knowledge about apoproteins is very vital in development of various lipid lowering medications.

Lipoproteins are mainly classified to five groups based on their density. They are described in the box.

Classification of Lipoproteins

Chylomicrons They are the largest lipoprotein particles and are primarily comprised of triglycerides. They are produced in the gut from dietary fat and cholesterol. Chylomicrons are not routinely measured as part of patient's lipid profile because they disappear from blood within 12 to 14 hours of last meal.

Very low density lipoprotein (VLDL) They predominantly contains triglycerides and has lesser amount of cholesterol. When VLDL particles secreted into the blood, they undergo chemical reaction and lose majority of triglycerides component. Then they become intermediate density lipoprotein (IDL) and subsequently to low-density lipoprotein (LDL).

Intermediate density lipoprotein (IDL) IDL is a short lived lipoprotein formed from VLDL and is converted into low-density lipoprotein (LDL).

Low-density lipoprotein (LDL) These molecules carry the most amount of cholesterol among lipoproteins. Half of the available LDL is taken up by the liver and the rest by the peripheral tissue.

High density lipoprotein (HDL) HDL particles are produced in the liver and intestine. They serve as return delivery system for cholesterol from peripheral cells back to the liver. HDL also removes cholesterol molecules that are incorporated in atherosclerotic plaque within arterial walls. Since they cause reduction in circulating cholesterol, HDL particles are often termed as good cholesterol. It is also believed that HDL has antioxidant and anti-inflammatory properties that aids in controlling atherogenesis.

Box 10.1 Classification of lipoproteins

Apoproteins play a major role in interaction of lipid molecules especially in processes like atherosclerosis. A specific protein component called **apoproteins-B (apo-B)** that is associated with VLDL, IDL, LDL and LP(a) is believed to have a major role in causing atherosclerotic process in familial hypercholesterolemia.

Lipoprotein (a)

It is commonly known as **lipoprotein little a**, a *modified form of low-density lipoprotein*. Clinical significance of lipoprotein (a) or **Lp(a)** is that it is *structurally similar to* **Plasminogen,** which is a plasma proteins involved in clot destruction upon activation. **Lp (a)** *can competitively inhibit Plasmin* because of its structural similarity and impair its normal physiologic functions. Since Lp(a) incorporates itself into the atherosclerotic plaque, its function in presence of a blood clot at the site of atherosclerotic plaque rupture can be counter-productive for averting the occlusion of the vessel from thrombus formation.

Lp (a) is considered as *one of the genetic risk factor for development of cardiovascular disease*. None of the studies have

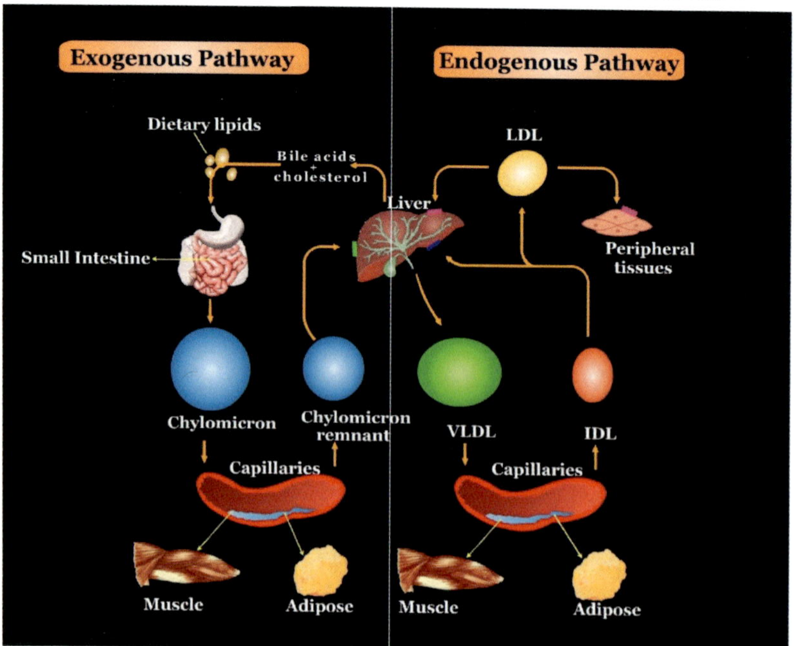

Fig 10.1 Lipoprotein synthesis

shown definite beneficial effect for aggressively lowering Lp(a) in patients with cardiovascular disease. **Nicotinic acid** is a drug proven to reduce lipoprotein (a) levels.

Serum lipoproteins are formed in two different pathways known as **exogenous pathway** (in the intestine through dietary intake) and **endogenous pathway** (from synthesis in the liver). These pathways are shown in the picture.

Dyslipidemia

Dyslipidemia is a disorder characterized by *abnormal amount of circulating cholesterol in the plasma*. It is established as one of the major risk factors for coronary artery disease. With advanced understanding of various aspects of lipoproteins and their effect in pathogenesis, **dyslipidemia** is differentiated into **hyperlipidemia** and **hypertriglyceridemia**. An abnormally low HDL can also be classified as dyslipidemia. The mechanism behind **dyslipidemia** can be genetic (**primary**) or external factors (**secondary**). However, in majority of patients with hyperlipidemia it is a mixture of both primary and secondary factors causing disease condition.

Secondary Causes of Dyslipidemia

Disease Conditions	Medications
• Diabetes mellitus • Chronic renal failure • Glomerulonephritis with nephrotic syndrome • Liver cirrhosis • Biliary obstruction • Hypothyroidism • Estrogen and progesterone	• Glucocorticoids • Thiazide diuretics • Non-selective beta-blockers • Anabolic steroids • Immunosuppressive agents • Anti-viral medications (HIV protease inhibitors)

Box 10.2 Secondary causes of hyperlipidemia

Genetic factors involving hyperlipidemia include mutation of apoproteins such as **apo B** leading to *impaired production and clearance of cholesterol*. Secondary factors are disease conditions like diabetes mellitus, obesity, lack of exercise, smoking, use of drugs such as beta-blockers and oral contraceptives.

Information from major epidemiologic studies like

ATP III Classification	
LDL cholesterol (mg/dl)	
<100	optimal
100- 129	near or above optimal
130 - 159	borderline high
160- 189	high
>190	very high
HDL cholesterol (mg/dl)	
<40	low
≥60	high
Total cholesterol (mg/dl)	
<200	desirable
200- 239	borderline high
>240	high

Table 10.1 ATP III risk assessment based on types of lipoproteins

ATP III recommendations for risk assessment	
CHD equivalents	**Major CHD risk factors**
• Diabetes mellitus • Symptomatic carotid artery disease • Peripheral artery disease • Abdominal aortic aneurysm • 10-year risk of CHD >20 %	• Cigarette smoking • Hypertension (>140/80 mm Hg or on antihypertensive drugs) • Low HDL cholesterol (<40 mg/dl) • Family history of premature CAD (in males first degree relative <55 yrs, in females first-degree relative <65 yrs) • Age (men ≥ 45 y, women ≥ 55 y) * HDL > 60 is a negative risk factor that takes one positive factor away from the total count

Box 10.3 Major Risk Factors for Coronary Heart Disease

Framingham heart study established the role of lipids among cardiovascular risk factors. **National cholesterol education program** (NCEP) developed the report on adult treatment plan for high cholesterol (**NCEP ATP III**) and it provides guidelines for maintaining various lipoprotein levels to reduce cardiovascular risk in patients with hyperlipidemia. One of such scoring system is called **Framingham risk score** that predict 10 years cardiovascular risk on an individual without known cardiovascular disease. **ATP III** guidelines for initiating treatment based on LDL-cholesterol level is shown in the Table.

Risk	LDL goal	Initiate TLC	Initiate drug therapy
0 or 1 risk factor	<160	≥160	≥190 (160-189 - optional drug therapy)
More than 2 risk factors			
10 yr risk <10%	<130	≥130	≥160
10 yr risk 10-20%	<130	≥130	≥130
CHD	<100	≥100	≥130
CHD risk equivalents 10 yr risk >20%	<70	≥100	≥130 (100-129 - optional drug therapy)
All units in mg/dL; CHD -Coronary heart disease; TLC- Therapeutic lifestyle changes			

Table 10.2 Treatment decision based on LDL-C level

Treatment of Hyperlipidemia

Patients who cannot achieve targeted LDL levels by therapeutic lifestyle changes (TLC) alone are treated with various forms of antilipidemic agents like **HMG-CoA reductase inhibitors** (**Statins**), **Nicotinic acid** (**Niacin**), **Cholesterol absorption inhibitors**, **Fibric acid derivatives** and **Bile acid resins**. This group of drugs and their examples are shown in the table.

HMG-CoA Reductase Inhibitors (Statins)

These are most commonly prescribed lipid-lowering medications because of their *potent LDL lowering capability*. The first agent among statins available for therapeutic use was **Lovastatin**. However in recent decades, there were a number of new agents came into the market having varying potency in their LDL lowering power. The effect of statins on various lipoproteins is shown in the table (Table 10.3).

> Along with their cholesterol lowering abilities, statins have secondary beneficial effects such as lowering risk of diabetes mellitus and reducing risk of osteoporosis especially in older patients. They also have minimal effect on lowering blood pressure in patients with hypertension.

Statins act by *inhibiting synthesis of cholesterol in the liver and enhancing reuptake of LDL cholesterol* (**LDL-C**) *from the blood*, thereby reducing the amount of circulatory lipoproteins especially LDL-C. They competitively inhibit **HMG-CoA reductase** involving with cholesterol synthesis in the liver. Enhancing number of LDL receptors in the liver for fast recycling of LDL-C from peripheral circulation also

Effects of Lipid-lowering Agents on Various Lipoproteins

Drug	Dosage®	Serum LDL	Serum HDL	Serum Triglycerides
Statins				
Pravastatin *Pravachol®*	10-40mg	↓22- 34 %	↑2-12 %	↓11 -24 %
Fluvastatin *Lescol®*	20-80 mg	↓22-36 %	↑ 3-6 %	↓12-18 %
Simvastatin *Zocor®*	20-80mg	↓24-40 %	↑7-16 %	↓12-21 %
Lovastatin *Mevacor®*	10-80 mg	↓ 24-48 %	↑7 %	↓ 10-14 %
Atorvastatin *Lipitor®*	10-80 mg	↓ 39-60 %	↑5-9 %	↓19-37 %
Rosuvastatin *Crestor®*	5-40 mg	↓ 47-65 %	↑2-9 %	↓ 20 %
Bile acid resins				
Cholestyramine *Questran®*	4-16gm	↓15-30 %	↑ 3-5 %	↑ 0-15* %
Colestipol *Colestid®*	Tab 2-16 gm Granules 5-30 gm			
Colesevelam *Welchol®*	3.75 gm			
Nicotinic Acid				
Niaspan®	1.5 -2 gm	↓12-21 %	↑18-30 %	↓15-44 %
Fibric acid derivatives				
Gemfibrozil *Lopid®*	600mg BID		↑6%	↓31%
Fenofibrate *Tricor®*	67-201 mg	↓ 20%	↑ 11%	↓ 38%
Cholesterol absorption inhibitors				
Ezetimibe *Zetia®*	10mg	↓16-19% ↓ 33-60%**	↑ 3-4% ↑ 8-11%**	↓ 5% ↓ 19-40 %**
Omega 3 fatty acid				
Loveza®	4 gm	↑ 4-49 %	↑ 5-9%	↓ 23 -45%

* in patients with underlying hypertriglyceridemia; ** When used with statins; ®Dosages are daily unless specified

Table 10.3 Effects of Lipid-lowering agents on various lipoproteins

results in increased uptake of **VLDL** and **IDL**.

Statins also cause *slight increase in* **HDL cholesterol** (**HDL-C**). Studies have shown that statins work in the form of '**anti-inflammatory agents**' by lowering **C-reactive protein** (**CRP**) levels and reducing inflammatory process in the atherosclerotic plaque. This action of statins is responsible for their plaque stabilization effect and thereby lowering incidence of acute plaque rupture. The effect of statins in plaque stabilization, reversal of endothelial dysfunction, decreased thrombogenicity, and reduced inflammation are known as **pleiotropic effects**. **Rosuvastatin** (**Crestor**) is one of the newer statins proven to *cause regression of atherosclerotic plaque*.

Majority of patients tolerate these medicines without having significant side-effects. However in a small percentage of population, statins can cause gastrointestinal upsets and headache. **Statins induced myopathy** is manifested with symptoms ranging from *reversible muscle pain and weakness to severe elevation in* **Creatine Kinase** (**CK**), leading to **Rhabdomyolysis** and **acute renal failure**. Incidence of statins induced myopathy is relatively low and in the order of 0.5%. Myopathy is diagnosed when patient has clinical symptoms of unusual muscle pain and weakness with Creatine phosphokinase (CK) level >10 times the upper limit of normal. Patients who are *susceptible for statins induced myopathy* are those with *renal failure*, *obstructive liver disease*, *hyperthyroidism*, *on treatment with* **Gemfibrozil**, **Cyclosporine** etc. Statins can also Increase liver enzymes without any associated symptoms. They should be *used with caution in patients with heavy alcohol use*.

> Many of the statins have short half-lives and are instructed to consume in the evening because the peak effect of these drugs will coincide with significant cholesterol production that happens in the body while the person is sleeping. Exceptions are Rosuvastatin and Atorvastatin, with longer half-lives.

Bile Acid Binding Resins

Bile acid binding resins are used as an *adjunct treatment in patients with hyperlipidemia* from elevated LDL levels. These agents work through the **exogenous pathway** of lipoprotein transport where they *decrease cholesterol absorption in the intestine* through enterohepatic circulation. These drugs are *not absorbed systemically* and create an insoluble compound with bile acids, which later excreted through feces. The reduction in cholesterol through enterohepatic circulation results in stimulation of more LDL receptors in the liver, which in turn increase reabsorption of circulating LDL cholesterol. The net effect is reduction in amount of circulating LDL-C.

However, during this process bile acid binding resins can *increase triglyceride levels* and therefore *should not be used in patients with elevated baseline hypertriglyceridemia*. These agents are **contraindicated** *in patients with biliary obstruction and chronic constipation*. Most common **side effects** *are gastrointestinal discomfort including flatulence*, *abdomen pain*, *bloating* and *heartburn*. Examples are **Cholestyramine** (**Questran®**), **Colestipol** (**Colestid®**) and **Colesevelam** (**Welchol®**). Since bile acid binding resins inhibit the absorption of cholesterol from the intestine, they need to be taken along with meals for maximum effectiveness.

> While taking bile acid binding resins, patients are instructed to take other medications especially thyroid hormones, antibiotics etc. at least one hour before or four hours after taking these agents because of their potential to bind with other drugs and interfere with their absorption. Patients should avoid taking bile acid resins with carbonated beverages as it may increase gastrointestinal upset.

Niacin

Nicotinic acid (**Niacin**) is a **naturally occurring vitamin B**, effective in reducing total cholesterol and triglyceride levels with *substantial improvement in HDL-C*. Effective dose of niacin is approximately 2 to 3 gm per day. Despite the excellent profile for improvement in HDL, many *patients cannot tolerate the required dose of Niacin* because of its annoying side-effects including *flushing* and *gastritis*. The symptoms of flushing can be avoided by taking **Aspirin** prior to Niacin intake or taking long acting slow-release preparation instead of short-acting Niacin.

Because of their side effect of having **hyperuricemia**, Niacin is generally contraindicated in patients with **gout**. Niacin is also **contraindicated** in patients with *severe hypotension*, *hepatic dysfunction* and *active peptic ulcers*. Niacin can also produce **Acanthosis nigrans** (hyper pigmentation of the skin). When used along with statins, liver function should be monitored periodically.

Some recent studies have shown that in patients with optimized statins therapy, **extended-release Niacin** may not provide any reduction in risk of cardiovascular disease however, can produce serious side effects like new onset diabetes, gastrointestinal or intracranial hemorrhage etc.

Cholesterol Absorption Inhibitors

Ezetimibe (**Zetia**) is the only member of cholesterol absorption inhibitor group with a unique mechanism of *selectively inhibiting cholesterol absorption* from the brush border cells of small intestine. This in turn reduces hepatic cholesterol reserve and thereby increases the reuptake of circulating lipoproteins. It can be *used either as mono therapy or as an adjunct for statins*. Ezetimibe has favorable effect on reducing total serum cholesterol, LDL- C, triglycerides and slightly increasing serum HDL-C. This agent is particularly useful in patients whose cholesterol numbers are not up to the goal either with high-dose statins or are unable to tolerate high doses of statins.

Fibric Acid Derivatives

Because of the beneficial action on triglycerides, Fibric acid derivatives are used for treatment of **high serum triglycerides**. They may *reduce serum triglycerides by 30 to 40%* and can *raise serum HDL by 10 to 15%*. They stimulate **lipoprotein lipase activity** that enhances triglycerides clearance. They also cause a shift of small dense LDL-C particles to less dense LDL -C, which has lower atherogenic capacity.

Major side effects of Fibric acid derivative group of drugs are *gastrointestinal intolerance* and an *increased risk of cholilithiasis*. Therefore, these agents are **contraindicated** in patients with a history of *gallstones and those with severe hepatic or renal dysfunction*. **Gemfibrozil** (**Lopid®**) **and Fenofibrate** (**Tricor®**) are the two agents available for therapeutic use. Among these, **Gemfibrozil** *along with* **Statins** or **Niacin** *may increase the chance of myopathy*. In order to avoid hepatotoxicity, liver function test (LFT) should be performed periodically. Elevation of LFT up to 2 to 3 times the upper normal limits may signal the need for discontinuation of Fibrates. It should also be *used with caution in patients taking anticoagulants* as it can increase the effect of anticoagulant like Coumadin.

Fish Oil

Fish oil contain polyunsaturated fatty acids like **Eicosapentaenoic acid** (**EPA**) and **Dicosahexaenoic acid** (**DHA**),

Drug	Onset/ peak**	Half Life	Metabolism	Elimination
Statins				
Pravastatin *Pravachol®*	Several days/ Peak 4 weeks	77 hrs	Hepatic	Feces and Urine
Fluvastatin *Lescol®*	Peak 4 weeks	2.5-2.8 hrs	Hepatic	Feces and Urine
Simvastatin *Zocor®*	> 3 days/ Peak 2 weeks	1.9 hrs	Hepatic	Feces and Urine
Lovastatin *Mevacor®*	3 days	1.1-1.7 hrs	Extensive first pass	Feces and Urine
Atorvastatin *Lipitor®*	3-5 days	20-30 hr	Hepatic	Bile and Urine
Rosuvastatin *Crestor®*	1 week	19 hrs	Hepatic	Feces
Bile acid resins				
Cholestyramine *Questran®*	21 days	Unknown	No systemic absorption	Feces
Colestipol *Colestid®*	24-48 hrs	Unknown	Not absorbed	Feces
Colesevelam *Welchol®*	2 weeks	Unknown	Not absorbed	Feces
Nicotinic Acid				
Niaspan®	30-60 min	20-45 min	Extensive first pass	Urine
Fibric acid derivatives				
Gemfibrozil *Lopid®*	Several days	1.5 hrs	Hepatic	Urine, Feces
Fenofibrate *Tricor®*	2-8 hrs	10-35 hrs	Hepatic	Urine and Feces
Cholesterol absorption inhibitors				
Ezetimibe *Zetia®*	4-12 hrs	22 hrs	Intestine and liver	Feces and Urine
** Onset and peak for therapeutic effect				

Table 10.4 Pharmacokinetics of lipid lowering agents

commonly known as **omega-3 fatty acids**. They *lower plasma triglyceride levels* and believed to have *antithrombotic properties*. Omega -3 fatty acids also *lower synthesis of VLDL*. For therapeutic purposes, omega-3 fatty acid preparations are *used for extreme hypertriglyceridemia*. There are number of studies in their active phase regarding the clinical influence of omega-3 fatty acid and its components, ranging from lowering triglycerides to their effect on blood pressure, vascular resistance, cardiac relaxation, antiarrhythmic and anti-inflammatory properties.

Points to remember!!!

- Cholesterol is an *essential component of cell membranes that helps in steroid hormone production and bile acid formation.*
- **Apolipoprotein** or apoproteins (**apo**) are specialized proteins that identify specific receptors to which the lipid particles interact.
- **Lipoprotein (a)** is commonly known as lipoprotein little a; a *modified form of low-density lipoprotein.*
- Clinical significance of lipoprotein (a) or **Lp (a)** is that it is *structurally similar to* **Plasminogen** which is a plasma proteins involved in clot destruction and therefore can cause thrombus burden in the arteries, leading to ischemic events.
- **Lp (a)** is considered as one *of the genetic risk factor for development of cardiovascular disease.*
- **Nicotinic acid** is a drug proven to reduce lipoprotein (a) levels.
- **Dyslipidemia** is a disorder characterized by *abnormal amount of circulating cholesterol in the plasma.*
- **Dyslipidemia** can be differentiated into **hyperlipidemia** and **hypertriglyceridemia**. An abnormally low HDL can also be classified as dyslipidemia.
- Genetic factors involving hyperlipidemia include mutation of apoproteins such as **apo B** leading to *impaired production and clearance of cholesterol.*
- Secondary factors are disease conditions like diabetes mellitus, obesity, lack of exercise, smoking, use of drugs such as beta-blockers and oral contraceptives.
- **HMG-CoA reductase inhibitors** (**Statins**) are most commonly prescribed lipid-lowering medications because of their *potent LDL lowering capability.*
- Statins may cause *slight increase in* **HDL cholesterol** (**HDL-C**) and work in the form of '**anti-inflammatory agents**' by lowering **C-reactive protein** (**CRP**) levels.

- The effect of statins in plaque stabilization, reversal of endothelial dysfunction, decreased thrombogenicity, and reduced inflammation is known as **pleiotropic effects**.

- **Rosuvastatin** (**Crestor**) is one of the newer statins proven to *cause regression of atherosclerotic plaque*.

- **Statins induced myopathy** is manifested with symptoms ranging from *reversible muscle pain and weakness to severe elevation in* **Creatine Kinase** (**CK**); leading to **Rhabdomyolysis** and **acute renal failure**.

- Incidence of statins induced myopathy is relatively low and in the order of 0.5%.

- Patients who are *susceptible for statins induced myopathy are those with renal failure, obstructive liver disease, hyperthyroidism, on treatment with* **Gemfibrozil**, **Cyclosporine** etc.

- Bile acid binding resins (e.g. **Cholestyramine (Questran®**) and **Colestipol** (**Colestid®**) and **Colesevelam** (**Welchol®**) are used as an *adjunct treatment in patients with hyperlipidemia* from elevated LDL levels.

- They work through the **exogenous pathway** of lipoprotein transport where they *decrease cholesterol absorption in the intestine* via enterohepatic circulation.

- Bile acid binding resins are *not absorbed systemically*.

- Bile acid binding resins can *increase triglyceride levels* and therefore *should not be used in patients with elevated baseline hypertriglyceridemia*.

- These agents are **contraindicated** *in patients with biliary obstruction and chronic constipation*.

- Most common **side effects** *are gastrointestinal discomfort including flatulence, abdomen pain, bloating* and *heartburn*.

- **Nicotinic acid** (**Niacin**) is a **naturally occurring vitamin B**, effective in reducing total cholesterol and triglyceride levels with *substantial improvement in HDL-C*.

- Many *patients cannot tolerate the required dose of Niacin* because of its annoying side-effects including *flushing* and *gastritis*.

- Because of their side effect of having **hyperuricemia**, Niacin is generally contraindicated in patients with **gout**.

- **Ezetimibe** (**Zetia**) is the only member of cholesterol absorption inhibitor group with a unique mechanism of *selectively inhibiting cholesterol absorption* from the brush border cells of small intestine. It is used either as mono therapy or as an adjunct for statins.

- Fibric acid derivatives (e.g. **Gemfibrozil (Lopid®) and Fenofibrate (Tricor®)** are used for treatment of **high serum triglycerides**.

- They may *reduce serum triglycerides by 30 to 40%* and can *raise serum HDL by 10 to 15%*.

- Major side effects of Fibric acid derivative group of drugs are *gastrointestinal intolerance and an increased risk of cholilithiasis*.

- **Gemfibrozil** *along with* **Statins** or **Niacin** *may increase the chance of myopathy*.

- **Gemfibrozil** can increase the effect of anticoagulant such as Coumadin.

- **Omega-3 fatty acids** lower *plasma triglyceride levels and believed to have antithrombotic properties*.

11 Nicotine and Other Cardiac Toxins

A number of chemical substances with high abuse potential are available to the general public that can produce serious cardiovascular complications. Nicotine, alcohol, cocaine, methamphetamine etc. are the prime suspects in acute and chronic cardiovascular diseases, especially in people without any other significant risk factors. Major chemicals and their cardiovascular effects are discussed here.

Nicotine

Cigarette smoking is one of the most common *preventable causes* of morbidity and mortality across the world. According to World Health Organization (WHO), at least 30% of cancer deaths, 80% of chronic obstructive pulmonary disease (COPD) related death and majority of early cardiovascular mortality are associated with tobacco dependence. The impact of cigarette smoking on society in general and health care in particular is so enormous that during recent decades consensus has been developed across various agencies in healthcare to effectively curb the dangers from tobacco dependence.

Across the world, tobacco is consumed in different forms like inhalation, sniffing and chewing. The rate of absorption and onset of action of **Nicotine**, which is the active ingredient of tobacco varies depending on the mode of ingestion. While smoking, the person is not only inhaling Nicotine, but also consuming many other toxic and carcinogenic substances such as carbon monoxide, formaldehyde, ammonia, arsenic and lead. Smoking has been identified as one of the major risk factor for development of early atherosclerotic disease through a number of epidemiologic studies. This highlights the importance of effectively addressing and treating patients with tobacco dependence to decrease cardiovascular morbidity and mortality.

Pathophysiology

Nicotine is the active chemical behind addiction from cigarette smoking. Nicotine is a *naturally occurring chemical neurotransmitter* in human beings. It has particular influence in physiologic functions like central and peripheral nervous system stimulation, respiratory stimulation, skeletal muscle relaxation, increasing blood pressure and heart rate, peripheral vasoconstriction etc. Activation of nicotine receptors in the brain produces *relaxation*, *increasing attention span*, *enhancement of learning* and *problem solving skills*. It also can cause weight loss and increases the risk of osteoporosis. Nicotine can affect **Cytochrome P450 system** (CYP 450) in the liver and can influence metabolism of many other drugs.

When absorbed from tobacco smoke, Nicotine transported through bloodstream from the pulmonary capillaries to the brain nicotine receptors in 10 to 15 seconds after the first puff. Nicotine has both *stimulant and depressant effect* on the brain. The stimulant effect of Nicotine is responsible for more alertness after smoking. Nicotine influences the **limbic system** of the brain that acts as '**reward system**', causing increase in **Dopamine,** that provides the person an urge to continue smoking in order to achieve this pleasurable state of mind.

Nicotine Withdrawal

Nicotine withdrawal is a sequela of nicotine dependent behavior. *Chronic use of nicotine results in an increase in number of nicotine receptors in the brain*. When the blood level of nicotine drops, chronic tobacco users starts having *irritability*, *restlessness*, *inability to concentrate*, *insomnia*, *depressed mood* etc. These are the typical symptoms of **nicotine withdrawal syndrome**. It is commonly seen upon sudden discontinuation of nicotine use in long-term tobacco users. The onset of the symptoms usually starts within 24 hours and can last for many days. Many of the pharmacologic agents used in treatment of smoking cessation are not only meant for smoking cessation, but also for prevention of

> While doing patient interview, it is important to assess the time when he or she likes their first cigarette of the day. Using cigarettes within '30 min of waking up' is one of the common sign of nicotine addiction.

withdrawal symptoms while the patient is in the process of quitting. The method for preventing withdrawal symptom is slow and gradual reduction in blood nicotine level.

Treatment of Nicotine Addiction

Like many other psychoactive substances producing addiction, Nicotine has both physiologic and psychologic components for its addictive behavior. Use of pharmaceutical agents to assist in 'quitting' may help very well with the physiologic part. However, the health care personal need to be mindful about providing enough psychologic support through behavioral modification, group therapy etc. for successful and lifelong smoking cessation.

Pharmacologic agents used in general for smoking cessation are either **controlled release Nicotine preparations** or **modulators of neurotransmitters** like Dopamine. In reality, many patients are treated with a combination of both of these agents to achieve higher level of success.

Nicotine Replacement Therapy

Controlled replacement of nicotine during smoking cessation phase can be achieved through various types of nicotine delivery systems like transdermal patch, inhaler, lozenges and nasal spray. It is vital to educate the patients who are making decision to quit by using any of these nicotine delivery product that the nicotine level from these drugs helps to avoid withdrawal symptoms, which is a common reason for patients to go back to smoking after quitting. These products do not deliver the same amount of nicotine as from a cigarette. These agents are generally contraindicated in patients with recent myocardial infarction coupled with life-threatening arrhythmia or worsening symptoms. Common forms of nicotine replacement therapy are explained in the box.

One of the major side effects with 24 hour Nicotine transdermal patch compared to its 16 hour counterpart is that the *24 hours patch may cause sleep impairment* because of its steady state of nicotine level during night. Local skin irritation is also reported as a side-effect and can be avoided by alternating the site of application of the patch. The patient should be weaned off of these patches by application of lower dose patches over time. Instruct the patient not to smoke while on transdermal patch

Nicotine Replacement Therapy

Nicotine gum (**Nicorette®**) This is a Nicotine resin complex, administered as 'chewing gum' over 30 min. Active nicotine is absorbed through oral mucosa. Chewing too quickly or smoking cigarette while chewing Nicotine gum can cause **Nicotine overdose** leading to *nausea*, *vomiting*, *headache* etc. Acidic foods like coffee and soft drinks can affect oral absorption of Nicotine and should be avoided 15 min before or after chewing the gum.

Nicotine lozenges Patients are instructed not to chew or swallow the lozenges since they have significant **first pass metabolism** upon ingestion which drastically reduce bioavailability of Nicotine. Similar to nicotine gum, these patients also should not be eating or drinking 15 min before or after having the product to facilitate effective absorption.

Nicotine transdermal patch (**Nicoderm CQ®**) This contains a nicotine reservoir shielded from patient's skin with a membrane that allows sustained release of the drug into the transdermal circulation. They are commonly used in everyday practice because of their ease of administration and better clinical profile. Transdermal system comes in 16 or 24-hour patches and are selected based on whether the patients have early morning withdrawal or craving symptoms. For chronic heavy smokers, early morning decline of nicotine in their blood cause withdrawal symptoms upon waking up, which lead to re-initiation of smoking behavior. These patients are treated with 24 hour patches that maintain blood nicotine level throughout night and especially in the early morning hours.

Nicotine spray and inhaler (**Nicotrol® Inhaler**) These are newer forms of nicotine delivery systems with relatively rapid onset of action and therefore particularly useful in patients with early morning withdrawal symptoms. It is important to monitor the amount of nicotine spray use in individual patients because of its 'potential for abuse'.

Box 11.1 Types of Nicotine replacement therapy

because of the *risk of myocardial infarction* or *life-threatening arrhythmia from Nocotine overdose*.

In the event of having toxicity symptoms like headache, nausea or vomiting, *the patch should be immediately discontinued*. However, because of the transdermal collection of nicotine, the drug delivery may continue for few more hours even after taking the patch off. Instruct the patients not to use soap on the site of patch application as it can increase absorption of remaining nicotine into

For patients treated with nicotine transdermal patch, symptom of delayed onset of sleep usually associate with a higher concentration or 'more than needed' nicotine dose. Similarly, early awakening suggest lack of enough dose causing withdrawal symptoms. Both require dose adjustments.

the bloodstream.

Neurochemical Modulators

These are pharmacologic agents mainly used for treatment of psychiatric disorders like depression. Even though several antidepressants are used successfully in treatment of smoking cessation, **Bupropion** (**Wellbutrin®, Zyban®**) which is a dopamine reuptake inhibitor is the only drug in this category approved by FDA as a smoking cessation aid. Its exact mechanism of action is still unclear however, its capacity to work as a **weak dopamine reuptake inhibitor** is believed to be the reason behind its pharmacologic action. Bupropion is started 1 to 2 weeks before 'quit smoking date' and continues for 7 to 12 weeks along with nicotine replacement therapy from the time of quitting. It is **contraindicated** in patients with *seizures*, *closed brain injury*, *history of stroke*, *anorexia or bulimia nervosa* and also *within 14 days of mono amine oxidase inhibitor* (MAOI) use. Common side effects of Bupropion are insomnia, dizziness, constipation and dry mouth.

A **partial agonist of nicotinic receptor** called **Varenicline** (**Chantix®**) is also used with success for smoking cessation. Along with its partial agonist action on the receptor, **Varenicline** has the unique property of **working as an antagonist in presence of nicotine**. This leads to prevention of withdrawal symptoms and helps to quit smoking. This drug causes higher incidence of cardiovascular events and therefore *used with caution in patients with history of cardiovascular disease*. It also has neuropsychiatric side effect profile and *may cause emotional lability*, *depression* and *suicidal thoughts*.

Cocaine

This is the most common illicit substance used by substance abusers that has a strong connection to serious cardiovascular disorders. Cocaine is widely popular because of the ease of administration, availability and low cost. The use of cocaine is also reinforced by the *misconception that recreational use of the drug does not possess the same toxicity as when used in higher doses*. Cocaine is extracted from the leaves of Coca plants, which is grown primarily in South America. There are two forms of cocaine available with distinct properties. **Cocaine hydrochloride** is a *water-soluble powder* and is used for *intranasal*, *intravenous* or *oral* consumption.

> Contrary to popular misconception, occurrence of myocardial infarction after cocaine use is unrelated to the amount of drug, route of administration or frequency of use.

The **freebase** form of cocaine is heat stable and is used for inhalation through smoking. This form of cocaine is also known as **crack cocaine** because of its *distinctive popping noise* while heating. This is the most potent and addictive form of cocaine with *onset of action within 3 to 5 seconds* upon inhalation and peak effect within 1 to 3 min. Serum half-life of cocaine is only 45 to 90 min and its metabolites can stay in blood up to 36 hours.

Cocaine is a powerful sympathomimetic drugs. This sympathetic nervous system activation is responsible for most of its clinical effects. Cardiovascular effects of cocaine include *increasing myocardial oxygen demand*, *marked arterial vasoconstriction*, *enhanced atherosclerosis*, *platelet aggregation* and *thrombus formation*. Among these, arterial vasoconstriction is significant on areas with underlying atherosclerotic disease. Therefore, in patients with underlying atherosclerotic heart disease, cocaine use may precipitate serious myocardial ischemic events.

Physiologic Effects of Cocaine

- Increase myocardial oxygen demand
- Profound arterial vasoconstriction
- Enhancing atherosclerosis
- Promoting platelet aggregation
- Facilitate thrombus formation

Box 11.2 Physiologic effect of Cocaine

Coronary vasospasm in cocaine use is believed to be due to the *stimulation of alpha adrenergic receptors* and is directly proportional to the serum concentration of the drug. In myocardial cells, cocaine acts as **sodium and potassium channel blocker**

Cocaethylene is an unique metabolite of cocaine, when used in conjunction with alcohol has lethal effect than cocaine alone. This is because of the synergistic effect with much potent sympathetic stimulation.

and thereby imparting effects of **class I anti arrhythmic agents**. Along with sympathomimetic activity, cocaine can induce lethal ventricular arrhythmias. Profound and repeated sympathetic activity induced by cocaine is similar to that of **pheochromocytoma**, which can lead to microscopic changes in the myocardium, resulting in **drug induced cardiomyopathy**. Cocaine can also *facilitate atherosclerotic and thrombus formation* by increasing endothelial permeability for LDL cholesterol. Subsequent structural defect in the endothelium leads to myocardial ischemia. Cocaine's ability to increase the concentration of **tissue plasminogen activator inhibitor** and enhancement of platelet aggregation result in formation of thrombus.

In some patients, cocaine use can produce *acute deterioration of left ventricular systolic and diastolic function* or transient '**ballooning**' of the apex of the heart called **Tako-tsubo cardiomyopathy** (meaning 'Octopus trap' in Japanese). This clinical condition is also seen especially in women who are experiencing severe emotional stress like loss of a family member and therefore is called **Broken heart syndrome**. It is purely a state of sympathetic over activity associated with underlying physical or emotional stress causing **reversible dilated cardiomyopathy.**

Amphetamine

Amphetamines were previously used for treatment of attention deficit disorder, obesity, nasal decongestion etc. However, because of their high abuse potential, the use of amphetamines nowadays is generally restricted . **Methamphetamine,** the common 'abuse drug' used as inhaled, smoked or injected form, is a **powerful sympathetic stimulant** with similar cardiovascular effect as that of cocaine.

Both cocaine and amphetamine produce a profound '***sense of well-being***' as part of their stimulant response. This euphoric feeling is responsible for the repeated use of these agents. They

Cardiovascular Effects of Cocaine and Amphetamine

- **Increase oxygen demand**

  Increase heart rate, contractility, arterial spasm, myocardial ischemia and infarction, Angina pectoris, systemic hypertension

- **Ventricular dysfunction**

  Ventricular hypertrophy, ventricular diastolic or systolic dysfunction, dilated cardiomyopathy

- **Arrhythmia**

  Prolong QRS and QT interval, Polymorphic ventricular tachycardia (Torsades de Pointes), Brugada type electrocardiogram

- **Other abnormalities**

  Endocarditis from intravenous use, Immunosuppressive effect, Aortic dissection due to acute hypertension

Box 11.3 Cardiovascular effect of Cocaine and Amphetamines

also inhibit reuptake of norepinephrine in the brain leading to enhanced arousal and vigilance. Cardiovascular effects of cocaine and amphetamine are described in the box.

A **synthetic Cathinone** with the street name ' **bath salt**' is a relatively new member of drugs with abuse potential, having similar pharmacologic effects as Amphetamine. It can also cause chest pain, palpitations and hypertension; however, does not appear to have pro-arrhythmic properties. Commonly it is produced from its precursor '**ephedrine**'. It is worth knowing that the name *bath salt* should not be confused with **Epsom salts** which is commonly used for regular water treatment purposes and does not possess any psychoactive properties.

Alcohol

Ethanol, the active ingredient of alcohol, has multitude of effect in myocardial structure and function. Being a chemical widely available for day-to-day use without much legal restrictions, alcohol involves with many cardiovascular disease processes when used in

Cardiovascular Effects of Alcohol

Functional impairment

- Left ventricular systolic dysfunction
- Left ventricular diastolic dysfunction
- Systemic arterial hypertension
- Increased risk for sudden cardiac death
- Development of arrhythmia (e.g. Atrial fib)

Structural impairment

- Myocardial fibrosis
- Development of atherosclerosis
- Increasing LDL and triglycerides

Box 11.4 ardiovascular effects of alcohol

excess. *Mild to moderate use of alcohol* (*3 to 9 drinks per week*) is generally considered to have beneficial effect for cardiovascular system especially in middle to old-age men who are otherwise healthy, compared to their younger counterparts. This beneficial effect is believed to be linked with *antioxidant*, *anti-inflammatory*, *antiplatelet*, and *fibrinolytic capabilities* of ethanol.

Unwanted cardiovascular effects of ethanol are contributed by factors like toxic metabolites (e.g. Acetaldehyde), associated electrolyte and vitamin imbalance (e.g. potassium, magnesium or thiamine deficiency) etc. Toxic impurities like lead and cobalt can also cause myocardial injury. **Myocardial fiber degeneration** and **subsequent fibrosis** occurs with continuous exposure to alcohol and its metabolites. Heavy alcohol consumption with *greater than six or more drinks per day* and *binge drinking* increase the risk of **sudden cardiac death** (**SCD**).

Binge alcohol drinking in otherwise healthy individuals of less than 65 years age happens especially during holidays and weekends; often cause development of **new onset of atrial fibrillation** and is called ' **Holiday heart syndrome**'. The treatment for ethanol induced atrial fibrillation is '**abstinence from alcohol**'.

Caffeine

Even though not considered as an 'abused drug' by general public, caffeine is the most widely used stimulant in the entire world. Caffeine and other Methylxanthines are the common ingredient of coffee, tea, cola, chocolate and energy drinks. Depending on the characteristics of coffee bean and brewing techniques, caffeine content from individual drink can vary considerably. Caffeine has 100% bioavailability. Contrary to the popular belief, *there is no scientific proof that regular amount of coffee consumption causes arrhythmias*. However, unusually large quantities of coffee consumption may precipitate caffeine toxicity with pro arrhythmic tendency. No studies have concluded with definitive evidence regarding the role of coffee in hypertension, cardiovascular disease, stroke etc.

Marijuana

Also known as **Cannabis**, is derived from cannabis plant and is used as a psychoactive substance. Even though it's medical use is controversial, *cannabis is used for treatment of nausea and vomiting associated with chemotherapy and as an analgesic*. Cardiovascular effects of cannabinoids results from **increase in sympathetic activity** and **decrease in parasympathetic response,** leading to tachycardia and enhanced cardiac output. However, in *higher doses marijuana inhibits sympathetic activity and increase parasympathetic response*, promoting bradycardia and hypotension. Smoking marijuana in patients with underlying coronary artery disease is high risk because of transient increase in myocardial oxygen demand secondary to tachycardia and increase in cardiac output.

Heroin

Heroin is a *derivative of morphine* and is the opioid most commonly used for abuse through injection. Synthetically, heroine is diacetylmorphine, also known in its street names as '*dope, smack, horse and tar*'. It can be used through intranasal, intravenous and inhalation routes. *Heroin is more lipid soluble than other opioids and therefore immediately crosses the blood brain barrier* and cause euphoric effects. Overdose of heroin can cause bradycardia and hypotension through increased parasympathetic activity. Enhanced automaticity in the myocardial cells can cause arrhythmia including ventricular tachycardia. Contaminated doses of the heroin with **Clenbuterol** a beta-2 agonist that occasionally used as a performance enhancement drug can cause tachycardia. Respiratory depression and non-cardiogenic pulmonary edema are possible outcome of heroin overdose.

Points to remember!!!

- Cigarette smoking is one of the most common *preventable causes* of morbidity and mortality across the world.

- Activation of nicotine receptors in the brain produces *relaxation, increasing attention span, enhancement of learning* and *problem solving skills*.

- Nicotine influences the **limbic system** of the brain which acts as '**reward system**'; causing increase in **Dopamine,** that provides the person an urge to continue smoking

- **Nicotine withdrawal syndrome** is manifested by *irritability, restlessness, inability to concentrate, insomnia, depressed mood* etc. It is commonly seen upon sudden discontinuation of nicotine use in long-term tobacco users.

- Pharmacologic agents used in general for smoking cessation are either **controlled release Nicotine preparations** or **modulators of neurotransmitters** such as Dopamine.

- *24 hours Nicotine patch may cause sleep impairment* because of its steady state of nicotine level during night.

- Instruct the patient not to smoke while on transdermal patch because of the *risk of myocardial infarction* or *life-threatening arrhythmia*.

- **Bupropion (Wellbutrin®, Zyban®)** which is a dopamine reuptake inhibitor is the only **Neurochemical Modulator** drug approved by FDA as a smoking cessation aid

- **Bupropion** is **contraindicated** in patients with *seizures, closed brain injury, history of stroke, anorexia or bulimia nervosa* and also *within 14 days of mono amine oxidase inhibitor* (MAOI) use.

- **Varenicline** has the unique property of **working as an antagonist in presence of nicotine**, leading to prevention of withdrawal symptoms

- **Cocaine hydrochloride** is a *water-soluble powder* and is used for *intranasal, intravenous* or *oral* consumption.

- The **freebase** form of cocaine (also known as **crack cocaine)** is heat stable and is used for inhalation through smoking.

- Cardiovascular effects of cocaine include *increasing myocardial oxygen demand, marked arterial vasoconstriction* and *enhancing atherosclerosis, platelet aggregation* and *thrombus formation*.

- Coronary vasospasm in cocaine use is believed to be due to the *stimulation of alpha adrenergic receptors* and is directly proportional to the serum concentration of the drug.

- In myocardial cells, cocaine acts as **sodium and potassium channel blocker** and thereby imparting effects of **class I anti arrhythmic agents**.

- Profound and repeated sympathetic activity induced by cocaine is similar to that of **pheochromocytoma**, which can lead to microscopic changes in the myocardium leading to **drug induced cardiomyopathy**.

- **Methamphetamine** which is the common 'abuse drug' used as inhaled, smoked or injected form; is a **powerful sympathetic stimulant** having similar cardiovascular effect as that of cocaine.

- *Mild to moderate use of alcohol* (*3 to 9 drinks per week*) is generally considered to have beneficial effect for cardiovascular system especially in middle to old-age men who are otherwise healthy

- **Myocardial fiber degeneration** and **subsequent fibrosis** occurs with continuous exposure to alcohol and its metabolites.

- Heavy alcohol consumption with *greater than six or more drinks per day* and *binge drinking* increase the risk of **sudden cardiac death (SCD)**.

- Contrary to the popular belief, *it has not been scientifically proven that regular amount of coffee consumption causes arrhythmias*.

- Cardiovascular effects of cannabinoids results from **increase in sympathetic activity** and **decrease in parasympathetic response** leading to tachycardia and enhanced cardiac output.

- In *higher doses, marijuana inhibits sympathetic activity and increase parasympathetic response*, promoting bradycardia and hypotension.

- Smoking marijuana in patients with underlying coronary artery disease is high risk because of transient increase in myocardial oxygen demand secondary to tachycardia and increase in cardiac output.

- Heroin is a *derivative of morphine* and is the opioid most commonly used for abuse through injection.

- *Heroin is more lipid soluble than other opioid and therefore immediately crosses the blood brain barrier* and cause euphoric effects.

- Overdose of heroin can cause bradycardia and hypotension through increased parasympathetic activity. It can also cause arrhythmias due to increased automaticity.

12 Pulmonary Hypertension and Other Vascular Disorders

Pulmonary Hypertension

Pulmonary arterial hypertension (**PAH**) is a progressive and fatal disease if left untreated. It is defined as the *abnormal and sustained elevation of mean pulmonary artery pressure greater than 25 mmHg at rest*. Elevated pulmonary vascular resistance eventually creates added stress to the right ventricle, leading to clinical manifestations like pulmonary congestion and right ventricular failure. **Cor pulmonale** is the right ventricular enlargement secondary to any underlying cardio-pulmonary disease process. Pulmonary hypertension is the most common cause of cor pulmonale.

From pathophysiologic point of view, consistent elevation of pulmonary artery pressure causes right ventricular remodeling to accommodate the back up of blood volume from the pulmonary circulation. Unlike left ventricle, *right ventricle only has a limited ability to accommodate the changes*, *leading to the dilation and eventual failure*. Most common cause of death in patients with pulmonary hypertension is the right heart failure.

In general, pulmonary hypertension is classified into five groups based on the underlying etiology as explained in the box. Among these, group 1 or pulmonary arterial hypertension is also known as **primary pulmonary hypertension** whereas, the rest of disorders come under **secondary pulmonary hypertension**.

True intention of treatment in pulmonary hypertension (PH) is to *treat underlying causative factors along with treatment of pulmonary hypertension proper*. Most common clinical presentations of pulmonary hypertension are exertional dyspnea, fatigue and peripheral edema. In advanced stages, exercise induced chest pain, syncope etc. may also develop. Hemoptysis and hoarseness of voice may rarely seen. Diagnosis of pulmonary

Classification of Pulmonary Hypertension

1. Pulmonary arterial hypertension (PAH)

Also known as Idiopathic pulmonary arterial hypertension (IPAH) caused by congenital heart disease, HIV infection, portal hypertension, chronic hemolytic anemia, drug and toxin (Fenfluramine, amphetamine, cocaine, chemotherapeutic agents, SSRI etc.).

2. Pulmonary hypertension due to left heart failure

PAH from systolic, diastolic and valvular heart disease.

3. Pulmonary hypertension from lung disease or hypoxia

COPD, interstitial lung disease, obstructive sleep apnea, alveolar hyperventilation disorders, chronic high-altitude exposure, developmental abnormalities.

4. Pulmonary hypertension from chronic thromboembolism

5. Pulmonary hypertension with unclear etiology

Hematologic disorders, systemic disorders (sarcoidosis), metabolic disorders (glycogen storage disease, thyroid disorders), tumor obstruction, chronic renal failure etc.

Box 12.1 Classification of Pulmonary Hypertension

hypertension is often delayed in patients with COPD because of the similar symptoms from underlying COPD. Echocardiogram, pulmonary function test and right heart catheterization provide definitive evidence for diagnosis of pulmonary hypertension.

Depending on the underlying pathology, patients may need primary or advanced therapy. All groups of patients require **primary therapy** with the use of *diuretics*, *anticoagulation* (*due to high risk of pulmonary embolism*), *continuous oxygen*, *exercise training* etc. **Digoxin** appears to be helpful in improving right ventricular ejection fraction in patients with COPD and biventricular failure. **Advanced therapy** for pulmonary hypertension is directed towards management of pulmonary hypertension itself rather than the underlying or associated factors. Advanced therapy is also indicated for patients who are either refractory to other treatment modalities or with advanced symptoms as per **World Health Organization** (**WHO**) **functional classification** as shown in the box.

Before initiating advanced therapy, these patients undergo invasive hemodynamic assessment for measuring reactivity of

WHO Functional Classification for PAH	
Functional class	**Characteristics**
Class I	Ordinary physical activity does not cause symptoms
Class II	Stable at rest; however, ordinary physical activity cause symptoms
Class III	Less than ordinary physical activity cause symptoms
Class IV	Symptoms even at rest

Box 12.2 WHO functional classification for PAH

pulmonary vasculature. **Vasoreactivity test** is done by *measuring the changes in pulmonary artery pressure in response to vasodilators such as* **intravenous adenosine**, **Epoprostenol** (**Flolan®**) or inhalation of **nitric oxide**. Vasoreactivity test is generally *considered positive if there is a drop in mean pulmonary pressure by 10 mmHg or to a value less than 40 mmHg*. Patients with idiopathic pulmonary artery hypertension (IPAH) are most likely to respond to vasoreactivity testing.

In patients with positive vasoreactivity test, trial of calcium channel blockers especially **Diltiazem** or **long acting Nifedipine** has shown survival benefit and functional improvement. In advanced functional class pulmonary hypertension, combinations of different agents from advanced therapy options are also being used. Definitive treatment for refractory pulmonary hypertension with debilitating symptoms is **lung transplant**.

Major components of advanced therapy in pulmonary hypertension are explained below.

Prostanoids

Prostanoids are members of the prostaglandin family including **Epoprostenol** (**Flolan®**), **Treprostinil** (**Remodulin®**) and **Iloprost** (**Ventavis®**), that are effective vasodilators. Among these, **Iloprost** is a *synthetic Prostacyclin analogues* used in intravenous, subcutaneous or by inhalation forms whereas the other two agents are used the form of continuous infusion through portable infusion pump. The pharmacologic characteristics and preferred indications of these agents are shown in the table (Table 12.1).

Endothelin Receptor Antagonists

Endothelin-1 is a potent vasoconstrictor that is seen in abundance during pulmonary hypertension. Endothelin receptor antagonists such as Bosentan **(Tracleer®)**, Ambrisentan **(Letairis®)** and Sitaxsentan **(Thelin®)** are proven to improve exercise tolerance, quality of life and hemodynamics in patients with pulmonary hypertension. Among these, **Ambrisentan (Letairis®)** and **Sitaxsentan (Thelin®)** are selective endothelin-1 receptor antagonists. **Sitaxsentan (Thelin®)** is no longer available worldwide secondary to severe hepatotoxicity, a common side-effect of all endothelin receptor antagonists. Because of the *high side-effect profile including teratogenicity and hepatotoxicity*, *this group of drug is of restricted use in United States*. All of these agents are metabolized via hepatic CYP450 enzyme system.

Treatment of Pulmonary Hypertension

Drug	Route	Onset	Half life	Indication
Prostanoids				
Epoprostenol *Flolan®*	Continuous IV	Immediate	6 min	• Primary PAH • Vasoreactivity testing • Intra-operative PAH during cardiac surgery** • Functional class IV *
Treprostinil *Remodulin®*	Continuous SubQ /IV	Immediate	4 hrs	• Primary PAH • Functional class IV
Iloprost *Ventavis®*	Inhaled			• Primary PAH • Functional class III/ IV*
Endothelin Receptor Antagonists				
Bosentan *Tracleer®*	Oral	3-5 hrs	5hrs (prolonged with CHF)	• Primary PAH • Functional class III/IV*
Ambrisentan *Letairis®*	Oral	2 hrs	9 hrs	• Primary PAH • Functional class III*
PDE-5 Inhibitors				
Sildenafil *Revatio® Viagra®*	Oral	60 min	four hours	• Functional class II /III* • Erectile dysfunction
Tadalafil *Cialis®*	Oral	60 min	15-17.5 hrs	• Functional class II/III * • Erectile dysfunction

** Off label use; * WHO Functional classification; CHF- congestive Heart Failure

Table 12.1 Treatment of Pulmonary hypertension

PDE-5 Inhibitors

Commonly used for treatment of erectile dysfunction, members of PDE-5 inhibitors such as **Sildenafil** **(Viagra®, Revatio®)**, **Tadalafil** **(Cialis®)** and **Vardenafil** **(Levitra®)** are utilized in management of pulmonary hypertension because of their vasodilatory effects. All of these agents are having beneficial effect in patients with primary pulmonary hypertension by improving functional capacity and hemodynamics.

Peripheral Vascular Disease (PVD)

Chronic diseases like diabetes mellitus, hypertension, hyperlipidemia and smoking are the primary risk factors for development of peripheral artery disease. Aggressive risk factor reduction and percutaneous catheter-based atherectomy treatments are the mainstay of management in these clinical situations. However, **Cilostazol** (Pletal®) and **Pentoxifylline** (Trental®) are two pharmacologic agents used in treatment of intermittent claudication associated with peripheral artery disease.

Among these, Cilostazol is primarily an *antiplatelet agents* under the category **Phosphodiesterase-3 Enzyme Inhibitor**. It also causes vasodilatation and inhibition of vascular smooth muscle cell proliferation. It is commonly used in combination with aspirin or Clopidogrel. **Pentoxifylline** is a **Xanthine** derivative, functions through reduction of blood viscosity by increasing flexibility of leukocytes and red blood cells. This reduction in blood viscosity helps to enhance blood flow and thereby improving peripheral tissue oxygenation. On an off label basis, Pentoxifylline is used for *treatment of venous leg ulcers*. Because of its potential **anti-tumor necrosis factor** (anti-TNF) property in management of inflammation, Pentoxifylline is used in treatment of severe **alcoholic liver disease.**

Drug	Onset/ peak	Half Life	Metabolism	Elimination
Cilostazol *Pletal®*	2-4 Wks**	11-13 hrs	Hepatic	Urine and Feces
Pentoxifylline *Trental®*	2-4 hrs	1.5 hrs	Hepatic	Urine

** For optimal therapeutic response

Table 12.2 Pharmacokinetics of PVD agents

Points to remember!!!

- **Pulmonary Hypertension** is defined as the *abnormal and sustained elevation of mean pulmonary artery pressure greater than 25 mmHg at rest.*

- **Cor pulmonale** is the right ventricular enlargement secondary to any underlying cardio-pulmonary disease process.

- Group 1 or pulmonary arterial hypertension is also known as **primary pulmonary hypertension** whereas the rest of disorders come under **secondary pulmonary hypertension**.

- All groups of patients require **primary therapy** with the use of *diuretics, anticoagulation* (*due to high risk of pulmonary embolism*), *continuous oxygen, exercise training* etc.

- **Advanced therapy** for pulmonary hypertension is directed towards management of pulmonary hypertension itself rather than the underlying or associated factors.

- **Vasoreactivity test** is done by *measuring the changes in pulmonary artery pressure in response to vasodilators such as* **intravenous adenosine**, **Epoprostenol** (**Flolan®**) or inhalation of **nitric oxide**.

- In patients with positive vasoreactivity test, trial of calcium channel blockers especially **Diltiazem** or **long acting Nifedipine** has shown survival benefit and functional improvement.

- Definitive treatment for refractory pulmonary hypertension with debilitating symptoms is **lung transplant**.

- Prostanoids are members of the prostaglandin family including **Epoprostenol** (**Flolan®**), **Treprostinil** (**Remodulin®**) and **Iloprost** (**Ventavis®**); that are effective vasodilators.

- **Endothelin receptor antagonists** such as **Bosentan (Tracleer®), Ambrisentan (Letairis®)** and **Sitaxsentan (Thelin®)** are proven to improve exercise tolerance, quality of life and hemodynamics

- Severe hepatotoxicity is a common side-effect of all endothelin receptor antagonists and therefore ***Endothelin receptor antagonists*** *group of drugs are of restricted use in United States.*

- PDE-5 inhibitors such as **Sildenafil (Viagra®, Revatio®), Tadalafil (Cialis®)** and **Vardenafil (Levitra®)** are utilized in management of pulmonary hypertension because of their vasodilatory effects

- **Cilostazol** (Pletal®) and **Pentoxifylline** (Trental®) are two pharmacologic agents used in treatment of intermittent claudication associated with peripheral artery disease.

- Cilostazol is primarily an *antiplatelet agent* under the category **Phosphodiesterase-3 Enzyme Inhibitor** and is capable of vasodilatation and inhibition of vascular smooth muscle cell proliferation.

- **Pentoxifylline** is a **Xanthine** derivative; functions through reduction of blood viscosity by increasing flexibility of leukocytes and red blood cells.

13 Antiarrhythmics

The contractile function of myocardium is a complex process involving electrical, chemical and mechanical coordination at the cellular level. Majority of these functions are modulated by movement of charged ions like Sodium, Potassium, Calcium, Chloride etc. across the cell membrane. A visual representation of the ionic transport at various phases of cardiac action potential is known as **cardiac action potential curve**.

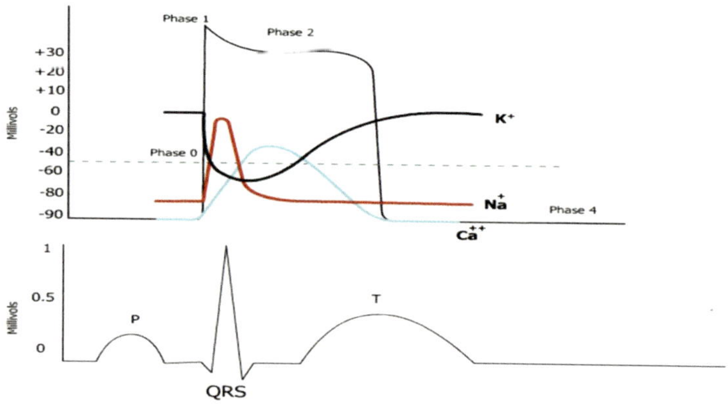

Fig 13.1 Action potential curve and ionic movements

Treatment of cardiac arrhythmias involves the use of various anti arrhythmic drugs, radiofrequency ablation of electrical pathways, surgical procedures and implantation of pacemakers and defibrillators. Among these, most common and least invasive treatment option is that of the pharmaceutical agents. Therefore, antiarrhythmic drugs play the major role of the treatment of common arrhythmias.

Classification of Antiarrhythmic Drugs

Common antiarrhythmic agents are generally classified

based on the pharmacodynamics by **Vaughan Williams classification**. However, many of these agents have multiple pathways for mechanism of action and can overlap between the classified groups. *Electrophysiologic effects of antiarrhythmic agents depend on the type of the tissue*, *membrane potential*, *heart rate*, *genetic variations*, *age* etc. Vaughan Williams classification therefore only provides a bird's eye view of the overall categorization of antiarrhythmic drugs based on their function at various levels of cardiac action potential curve.

Based on the electrical ion they regulate, antiarrhythmic drugs are generally classified into four groups. Class **I** agents are **sodium channel blockers**, **Beta-blockers** in class **II**, **Potassium channel blockers** in class **III** and **Calcium channel blockers** in class **IV**. Adenosine and Digoxin are classified as class **V** in this system.

Class I Antiarrhythmic Drugs

These agents are otherwise known as **Sodium channel blockers**. They control the *movement of sodium ions in phase 0* of cardiac action potential curve. By modulating sodium ions at this stage, these drugs can essentially influence the onset of cardiac

Classification of Antiarrhythmic Drugs

Class I		**Sodium channel blockers**
	Class IA	Procanamide Quinidine Disopyramide (*Norpace®*, *Rythmodan®*)
	Class 1B	Lidocaine (*Xylocaine®*) Mexiletine
	Class 1C	Flecainide (*Tambocor®*) Propafenone (*Rythmol®*)
Class II		**Beta-blockers**
		Carvedilol (*Coreg®*) Metoprolol (*Lopressor®*)
Class III		**Potassium channel blockers**
		Amiodarone (*Pacerone®*) Sotalol (*Betapace®*) Dronedarone (*Multaq®*) Ibutilide (*Corvert®*) Dofetilide (*Tikosyn®*)
Class IV		**Calcium channel blockers**
		Verapamil (*Calan®*) Diltiazem (*Cardizem®*)
Class V		**Other antiarrhythmics**
		Digoxin (*Lanoxin®*) Adenosine (*Adenocard®*)

Box 13.1 Classification of antiarrhythmic drugs

action potential. Depending on the ease of binding and dissociation with the receptor sites, they are further classified into class **1C** (having *slowest rate of binding and dissociation*), class **1B** (has *rapid binding and release*) and class **1A** (with *intermediate binding and dissociation*).

Since these agents vary in the rate of receptor attachment, it is of great use in managing both faster and slower rhythms. For example, class **1C** drugs (**Flecainide** and **Propafenone**) when used during fast heart rate, takes more time to dissociate from the receptor sites and make less number of receptors available for active contractile function. This effect essentially lowers the heart rate because of lack of resources to continue rapid action potential cycles. This property is called **use dependent channel block**. They primarily block sodium channels open for business and thereby slow the conduction.

Conversely, some drugs exert greater effects at slow heart rate than at the fast rate known as **reverse use dependent channel blockers**. When using these agents, *the QT interval becomes more prolonged at slow rather than fast heart rate*. They can potentially cause polymorphic ventricular tachycardia because of their QT prolongation at slow heart rate leading to prolonged refractoriness of the cells. The efficacy of sodium channel blocking property is *highest for class 1C drugs*, *followed by class 1A and class 1B (C-A-B)*.

Class 1A Antiarrhythmic Agents

Sodium channel blocking properties of these agents are *intermediate* to that of other subclasses of class **I** antiarrhythmics.

When using Class 1A agents *to treat atrial fibrillation or flutter*, *ventricular rate control with use of beta-blockers or calcium channel blocker is recommended*. This is because the reduction of atrial flutter or fibrillation rate caused by **Quinidine** coupled with its vagolytic effect on **AV node** can cause 1:1 ventricular response; leading to hemodynamic compromise. For example, with an original atrial rate of 300 bpm reduced to 200bpm by the use of Quinidine; an original 2:1 conduction (with an effective ventricular rate of 150 bpm with a 2:1 conduction) now become 1:1 conduction ratio(with an effective ventricular rate of 200 bpm).

Quinidine, **Procanamide** and **Disopyramide** are prime examples of this group. Among these, **Quinidine** has many drug-to-drug interactions especially when using with Verapamil, Phenytoin, Digoxin etc. Pro-arrhythmic effect of these medications can cause formation of **Torsades De Pointes** especially in patients with prolonged base line QT interval and electrolyte abnormalities. If the baseline *QTC is greater than 500 ms*, use of Class 1A antiarrhythmics are *cautioned*. Therefore, in susceptible patients initiation of these drugs requires *in hospital monitoring*. In general, all of these drugs can spare sinus node from any effect as long as it is healthy. When used for patients with sick sinus syndrome or any other sinus node dysfunction, class I drugs may increase sinus node recovery time.

Quinidine

Only in patients with *pre-existing sinus node dysfunction,* **Quinidine** *depresses sinus node automaticity*. It has significant anticholinergic effect and reflex sympathetic stimulation resulting from alpha blockade action, leading to peripheral vasodilation. Using Quinidine along *with other vasodilators may cause significant hypotension*. Quinidine prolongs repolarization and thereby QT interval, especially at slower heart rates (**reverse use dependent blockade**).

> **Quinidine** is derived from **Cinchona bark** and has properties of *antimalarial*, *antipyretic* and *vagolytic actions*.

Quinidine is particularly useful in *treatment of premature supraventricular and ventricular complexes*. It also *prevents spontaneous recurrence of AV nodal re-entry tachycardia* (AVNRT) by prolonging refractoriness of atrial and ventricular contraction in the re-entry circuit. Quinidine is also used for *termination of atrial flutter of atrial fibrillation* in new onset arrhythmia.

Most common side effects of oral Quinidine therapy are gastrointestinal origin including abdominal pain, nausea, vomiting and diarrhea. It can also cause delirium, hearing loss, confusion and psychosis. The *incidences of adverse events are up to 30 to 40%* in long-term therapy using Quinidine. Up to 2% of patients develop syncope episodes while on Quinidine mostly because of the Q-T prolongation property of this drug. *Intravenous magnesium is the treatment of choice for patients with* **Quinidine syncope**. Due to the high side effect profile and availability of better agents, Quinidine is not commonly used in current cardiology practice settings.

Procainamide

Similar to that of Quinidine, Procainamide exerts its effects through *reducing automaticity, conductivity and excitability of the conduction system*. It has least amount of anticholinergic effects among all the drugs in class **1A** and therefore *is better tolerated than Quinidine*. Procainamide is used for treatment of both *supraventricular and ventricular arrhythmias*. Like Quinidine, Procainamide is useful in *treatment of new onset atrial fibrillation or flutter*. Because of its effects on accessory pathway conduction, Procanamide is successful in treating *atrial fibrillation with WPW syndrome*. It can *cause significant bundle branch block* and therefore used with caution in patients with underlying Bundle of his and Purkinjee fiber disease. Similar to Quinidine, patients having *atrial fibrillation with rapid ventricular response should be treated with beta or calcium channel blockers prior to the use of Procanamide* to avoid ventricular tachyarrhythmia from possible 1:1 conduction through the AV node.

Common side effects from Procanamide treatment are *myalgia*, *Raynaud's phenomena*, *agranulocytosis*, *prolonged QT syndrome* leading to *polymorphic VT*. For patients with underlying sick sinus syndrome, Procanamide *can increase* **sinus node recovery time** and therefore chances of syncope. Chronic use of Procanamide can cause **systemic Lupus Erythematosis** (SLE) **like syndrome** characterized by *hepatomegaly*, *fever*, *arthralgia*, *pericardial effusion* or *cardiac tamponade*. This condition resolves with discontinuing Procanamide. Procanamide may *increase defibrillation threshold*.

Disopyramide (**Norpace®**)

Disopyramide is used for treatment of *recurrent ventricular tachycardia and atrial fibrillation*. It has greater anticholinergic effect than that of Quinidine. It prolongs both atrial and ventricular refractory period. Disopyramide has *negative inotropic effect in the ventricle* and therefore is not generally indicated for patients with reduced left ventricular function.

Disopyramide can cause *Q-T prolongation and polymorphic VT*. It can produce less serious side effects like urinary retention, constipation, dry mouth etc. that are characteristic anticholinergic symptoms. Disopyramide may also cause reduction in left ventricular contractility in patients with underlying left ventricular dysfunction as mentioned before.

Class IA Antiarrhythmics

Indication	Onset/ Peak	Half-life	Metabolism	Elimination	Contraindication	Side-effects
Quinidine						
• PSVT • PVC • New onset Atrial fib/flutter	2-3 hrs (PO)	6-8 hrs	Extensive hepatic	Urine	• Hypersensitivity • Thrombocytopenia • Sinus node dysfunction	• Hypotension • Q-T prolongation • Syncope • Diarrhea • Nausea and vomiting • Dizziness
Procainamide						
• New onset Atrial fib/flutter • Afib with WPW syndrome • Ventricular arrhythmia	10-30 min (IM)	2.5- 4.7 hrs	Hepatic	Urine and Feces	• Sick sinus syndrome • Complete heart block • Second-degree AV block without pacemaker	• Myalgia • Raynaud's phenomena • Agranulocytosis • Polymorphic VT • Prolong QT interval • SLE like syndrome
Disopyramide (Norpace®)						
• Sustained VT • Atrial fibrillation	0.5 to 3.5 hrs (PO)	4-10 hours	Hepatic	Urine and feces	• Heart block with order pacemaker • Congenital QT syndrome • Sick sinus syndrome	• Q-T prolongation • Polymorphic VT • Syncope • Dry mouth (Xerostomia) • Constipation

Table 13.1 Class IA antiarrhythmics

Class 1B Antiarrhythmic Agents

Lidocaine and **Mexiletine** are classified into class **1B** antiarrhythmics. They are particularly *useful in treating ventricular arrhythmias* in the setting of myocardial infarction due to their efficacy in *fast heart rate* and *in abnormal myocardium*.

Lidocaine

Lidocaine has *rapid onset and offset from its receptors*. It has extensive **first pass metabolism** in the liver, that reduces the availability of drug when taken orally. Therefore, Lidocaine should be administered intravenously. Lidocaine is particularly useful in treatment of *ventricular arrhythmias especially after coronary revascularization* and for patients *resuscitated after out-of-hospital ventricular fibrillation arrest*. Most common adverse effects of Lidocaine are dizziness, parasthesia, confusion, seizures etc. and are commonly dose-related. *Nystagmus* is a common early indication of Lidocaine toxicity. Lidocaine may *increase defibrillation threshold*.

Mexiletine

Mexiletine is useful for treatment of patients with *symptomatic ventricular tachycardia*. It is not effective in

Class IB Antiarrhythmics

Indication	Onset/ Peak	Half-life	Metabolism	Elimination	Contraindication	Side-effects
Lidocaine						
• Ventricular arrhythmias from myocardial infarction or revascularization	45-90 seconds (IV)	1.5-2 hours	Extensive hepatic	Urine	• Hypersensitivity • Sick sinus syndrome • WPW syndrome • Heart block	• Dizziness • Confusion • Seizures • Parasthesia • Increased defibrillation threshold (mostly dose related)
Mexiletine						
• Symptomatic ventricular tachycardia • Suppression of PVC	2-3 hours	10-14 hours	Hepatic	Urine	• Cardiogenic shock • Second or third degree AV block without a pacemaker	• Lightheadedness • Dizziness • GI distress • Nausea vomiting • Proarrhythmia

Table 13.2 Class IB antiarrhythmic agents

supraventricular rhythms. Mexiletine is used as an *oral equivalent* of Lidocaine in many situations. Compared to that of Lidocaine, Mexiletine has minimal hemodynamic effects. The side-effect profile of Mexiletine is similar to that of Lidocaine including dizziness, confusion, dyspepsia etc.

Class 1C Antiarrhythmic Agents

Flecainide and **Propafenone** are used for treatment of *atrial fibrillation*. Flecainide and Propafenone can cause harmful effects in patients *with structural heart disease* like prior history of myocardial ischemia or infarction and are generally *contraindicated* in these settings.

Flecainide (Tambocor®)

Because of the slow dissociation of Flecainide from sodium channels, significant effect of this drug is seen in lower heart rates (**reverse use dependence**). Flecainide is useful for treatment of *non-sustained ventricular tachycardia*, *atrial tachycardia*, *flutter* and *fibrillation*. Most important adverse effect of Flecainide is the *pro arrhythmic effect*. It can happen in up to 30% of patients especially *with underlying cardiac decompensation* and *ventricular arrhythmia*. Therefore, Flecainide is routinely initiated in hospital under continuous cardiac monitoring. *Negative inotropic effect exerted by this drug can worsen heart failure*. It can cause sinus node dysfunction and *increase pacing threshold*.

Propafenone (Rythmol®)

Like Flecainide, **Propafenone** is also used for treatment of *paroxysmal supraventricular tachycardia*, *atrial fibrillation* and ventricular arrhythmias, especially *non-sustained and sustained ventricular tachycardia*. It has *greater effect in the ischemic tissue than normal*. Propafenone is used with *caution in patients having severe left ventricular dysfunction* because of the negative ionotropic property. It decreases excitability and suppresses spontaneous automaticity. Therefore, Propafenone is effective in

> **Flecainide** and **Propafenone** are generally initiated in hospital setting with continuous cardiac monitoring because of the risk of ventricular arrhythmia.

Indication	Onset/ Peak	Half-life	Metabolism	Elimination	Contraindication	Side-effects
Flecainide (Tambocor®)						
• Paroxysmal supraventricular tachycardia • Atrial fibrillation • Non-sustained VT	1.5-3 hours	11-12 hours	Hepatic	Urine	• Pre-existing advanced heart block without pacemaker • Cardiac shock • Underlying structural heart disease	• Atrioventricular block • Worsening heart failure • Dizziness • Blurred vision
Propafenone(Rythmol®)						
• PSVT • Paroxysmal Afib	3.5 hrs	2-10 hours	Hepatic	Urine and feces	• Brugada syndrome • Sinus node dysfunction • Uncompensated heart failure • COPD and other bronchospastic disorders	• Proarrhythmic effect • Congestive heart failure • Dizziness • Unusual taste • Dyspnea

** Only used in the absence of structural heart disease

Table 13.3 Class IC antiarrhythmics

controlling spontaneous premature ventricular contractions, that acts as trigger for many arrhythmic episodes.

Propafenone may cause pro arrhythmic effects especially in patients with history of sustained ventricular tachycardia and left ventricular dysfunction. However, the *side-effect profile is better than that of Flecainide*. It can also cause *atrio ventricular block*, *worsening of heart failure* and less serious side effect like dizziness, blurred vision etc. Propafenone initiation can unmask underlying Brugada syndrome in otherwise asymptomatic patients.

Class II Antiarrhythmics

These agents are known as **Beta-blockers**, with the characteristic beta-adrenergic receptor blockade property. Depending on the lipid solubility and route of elimination, they have different plasma half-lives. For example, lipid soluble beta-blockers like Metoprolol and Propranolol metabolize through liver and have shorter half-life. However, Atenolol with prominent renal clearance stays in blood longer. Beta-blockers can be **selective beta I receptor blockers** (cardio selective) or **non-selective beta blockers** (non-

It is important to keep in mind that *beta 1 selectivity of Beta blockers only exist in lower doses*. At higher doses, even the selective beta-blockers affect both beta-1 and beta-2 receptors.

cardio selective). Since *beta-1 receptor blockers selectively influence the heart*, they are of greater use in clinical situations like bronchial asthma, where beta-2 receptors can cause adverse effects.

Beta blockers exert antiarrhythmic property through *suppression of arrhythmias resulting from autonomic nervous system stimulation*. In terms of pharmacodynamics, they counteract the effect of catecholamine at beta-adrenergic receptor sites. Resultant *decrease in contractility* (*negative ionotropic effect*) and slow heart rate by *reducing automaticity* (*negative chronotropic effect*) are the mechanisms behind their action. These agents are useful in treating both ventricular and atrial arrhythmia especially during *high catecholamine states like myocardial ischemia and perioperative stage*. Among these, **Sotalol** has more class **III** antiarrhythmic properties than beta blockade.

Beta-blockers are particularly useful in controlling arrhythmias associated with high catecholamine states like *thyrotoxicosis*, *pheochromocytoma* or those related with adrenergic stimulation from *exercise*, *emotions* or use of stimulants like *cocaine*. Because of the profound beta blocking effect on the atrioventricular node, these agents can *control ventricular rate in patients with atrial fibrillation*. Beta-blockers are also useful in *management of re-entry tachycardia* like AVNRT or those associated with WPW syndrome. Because of their lack of effect in the ventricular conduction system, beta-blockers are *useful in treating ventricular arrhythmias associated with prolonged QT interval*.

Beta-blockers slows sinus discharge rate and therefore can cause *significant bradycardia in patients with underlying sinus node dysfunction*. It does not affect the conduction and refractoriness of ventricular tissue evidenced by lack of any effect on QRS duration or QT interval.

The negative ionotropic and chronotropic effect of Beta blockers are responsible for adverse reactions like *hypotension, severe bradycardia and exacerbation of congestive heart failure* (in acute phase). For detailed explanations, please see chapter 3.

Class III Antiarrhythmics

This group of medications have characteristic **potassium channel blocking** properties. Exceptions are **Sotalol**, with *both beta blocking and potassium channel blocking* properties and **Amiodarone** with a wide range of properties extending from *class 1 to 4 effects*. These medications are particularly useful in atrial fibrillation, flutter and ventricular tachyarrhythmia. They cause *increase in duration of cardiac action potential* and therefore *prolong QT interval* in EKG.

Amiodarone (Pacerone®)

Amiodarone, being a major player in class III antiarrhythmic drugs has a wide range of use in both emergent and chronic situations. When given intravenously during an *acute myocardial event*, Amiodarone shows more of *class I* and *IV properties* (*sodium* and *calcium channel blocking*) and thereby effectively *treats faster ventricular arrhythmias*. When given *intravenously compared to oral route*, *Amiodarone can cause negative ionotropic effect* in the left ventricle. This may cause problems with patients having underlying LV dysfunction.

Amiodarone is used with varying levels of success in treatment of supraventricular and ventricular arrhythmias including *re-entry tachycardia*, *atrial flutter* and *fibrillation*, *ventricular tachycardia* or *fibrillation*. It is commonly used in patients post myocardial infarction and cardiac arrest to treat ventricular arrhythmias. Amiodarone is also useful in treating ventricular arrhythmias associated with hypertrophic obstructive cardiomyopathy (HOCM) and non-ischemic dilated cardiomyopathy. Amiodarone is *superior to class I antiarrhythmics and Sotalol in maintaining sinus rhythm* for patients with recurrent atrial fibrillation. Amiodarone can *reduce the incidence of spontaneous ventricular tachycardia* and resultant shock therapy in patients with implantable cardioverter defibrillator (ICD).

> Amiodarone is highly fat-soluble and takes many weeks before reaching steady state in the body. Because of this extensive fat solubility and distribution, it is *not dialyzable* and Amiodarone stays in body for longer duration (Up to 2 months). Amiodarone is predominantly *metabolized through the liver*.

There are varying degree of side effects mostly from chronic use of Amiodarone for up to 75% of patients including *chronic interstitial pneumonitis*, *thyroid dysfunction*, *photosensitivity*, *peripheral neuropathy* etc. Amiodarone must be discontinued in the event of pulmonary toxicity. Patients with long-term high-dose Amiodarone therapy are routinely tested with chest radiograph and pulmonary function test including carbon monoxide diffusion capacity (PFT with DLCO) for early detection of pulmonary complications. At lower maintenance doses, the chances of adverse side effects are minimal. Liver toxicity in the form of asymptomatic elevation of liver enzymes or fatal liver cirrhosis can also develop as a complication of long-term Amiodarone therapy. Amiodarone should be stopped in patients with 2 to 3 fold elevation of liver enzymes from baseline to prevent lethal toxic effects.

Unlike many other antiarrhythmic drugs such as Sotalol, Procanamide etc, Amiodarone *does not require hospitalization* for dose initiation because of its low propensity for producing **polymorphic VT** compared to other agents.

Baseline thyroid function should be tested to identify hypothyroidism in patients with long-term Amiodarone therapy. Thyroid dysfunction occurs because of the effect of Amiodarone in the thyroid tissue. High Iodine load from chronic Amiodarone use is also believed to have contributing effect on thyroid. Bradycardia, worsening of ventricular tachyarrhythmia including Torsades are also reported as side effects. Similar to many other antiarrhythmics, Amiodarone has pro-arrhythmic effect due to *Q-T prolongation*. It can also cause bradycardia, especially with concomitant use of Beta-blockers. In chronic use, Amiodarone has shown to increase **defibrillation threshold** (energy required for successful conversion of ventricular tachyarrhythmia). Amiodarone interacts with **Digoxin** and **Coumadin** and therefore requires careful *monitoring and dosage adjustments when used together*.

Dronedarone (Multaq®)

Dronedarone is indicated for *chemical cardioversion of atrial fibrillation or flutter* and *maintenance of sinus rhythm after conversion*. It is slightly less effective than Amiodarone however, because of the lack of iodine molecule, Dronedarone has a better side effect profile.In light of the higher mortality rate, Dronedarone is *contraindicated for use in patients with underlying advanced heart failure*. It is also contraindicated in patients with severe liver dysfunction. Dronedarone does not have the same pro arrhythmic effect like Amiodarone. Absence of iodine molecule is believed to be responsible for low incidence of lung and thyroid toxicity.

Sotalol (**Betapace®**)

Sotalol is a nonselective beta-blocker without intrinsic sympathomimetic activity. Sotalol is useful in treatment of *ventricular arrhythmias*, *atrial fibrillation* and other *supraventricular tachycardia*. This drug *prolongs atrial and ventricular depolarization* by extending the phase 2 (plateau phase) of the cardiac action potential through reducing outward movements of potassium ions. This action potential prolongation is predominantly seen in slow heart rate (**reverse use dependent**). In patients with underlying left ventricular dysfunction, Sotalol can cause reduction in cardiac index and increase in filling pressures leading to *exacerbation of heart failure*. Therefore, Sotalol must be used with caution in patients having underlying LV dysfunction.

Sotalol is *comparable to Amiodarone in effectiveness* for treatment of ventricular tachyarrhythmia and prevention of recurrent atrial fibrillation after cardioversion. It reduces ventricular response to atrial tachyarrhythmias. Side effects of Sotalol include *bradycardia,* due to beta blocking property and *Q-T prolongation* and *risk of polymorphic VT* (Torsades). The QT prolongation and risk of polymorphic VT are part of potassium channel blocking and reverse use dependence behavior. This can happen for up to 4% of patients.

> Sotalol should be *used with caution along with Class IA antiarrhythmics* (Quinidine, Procainamide and Disopyramide) because of their synergistic effect on refractoriness; leading to lethal ventricular arrhythmia.

Sotalol, having both beta blocking and potassium channel blocking properties, is widely used for management of *atrial fibrillation* especially in patients *with implantable defibrillator*. Unlike Amiodarone, *Sotalol reduces the defibrillation threshold*. Because of predominant renal clearance, Sotalol is *not ideal in renal dysfunction*. In patients with risk factors for polymorphic VT (Torsades), initiation of Sotalol should only be done under monitoring in the hospital.

Ibutilide (**Corvert®**)

Ibutilide is a class III potassium channel blocker administered intravenously and is used for *acute termination of established atrial fibrillation or flutter*. Since Ibutilide is only suitable for termination of atrial fibrillation rather than its prevention, it should not be given in patients with paroxysmal atrial fibrillation. Ibutilide has also proven to be effective for *pre-treatment of patients undergoing electrical cardioversion* to increase the likelihood of termination of atrial fibrillation. It does not have any significant hemodynamic side effects.

The most important and serious side effects of Ibutilide is the incidence of *Q-T prolongation and Torsades de Pointes*, that mostly occurs in 4 to 6 hours after administration of the drug. It happens in approximately 2% of population and the incidence are more in women. Ibutilide is *contraindicated* for patients with *QTc greater than for 440 ms in presence of hypokalemia*, *bradycardia* and *other QT prolonging drugs*.

Dofetilide (**Tikosyn®**)

Dofetilide is an oral class **III** antiarrhythmic agent used for both *conversion of atrial fibrillation* and *termination of recurrent episodes* of atrial fibrillation in long-term. The use and distribution of Dofetilide is restricted in United States and therefore specially certified practitioners can only write the prescription. *High incidence of Q-T prolongation and resultant Torsades de Pointes* is seen as a complication of Dofetilide. It does not have any significant hemodynamic effects. The patients should be hospitalized with continuous electrocardiogram monitoring when initiating and titrating this drug to detect any Q-T prolongation issues. The dosage should be titrated based on the QT interval. The effect of Dofetilide is more pronounced in atria than in ventricle. Therefore, Dofetilide is particularly useful in prevention of supraventricular tachycardia including atrial fibrillation and flutter. Like other potassium blocking antiarrhythmic agents, Dofetilide also cause increase in incidence of Torsades in presence of hypokalemia, baseline Q-T prolongation and QT prolonging drugs. Incidents of Torsade de Pointes are highest during first three days of drug initiation and requires close monitoring. *Renal impairment demands dose reduction* as this drug

Indication	Onset / Peak	Half-life	Metabolism	Elimination	Contraindication	Side-effects
Amiodarone						
• Ventricular tachycardia • Ventricular fibrillation • Atrial fib • Atrial flutter • Re-entry tachycardia • Paroxysmal SVT • Adjunct to ICD therapy	2-21 days	26-107 days (for elimination)	Hepatic (with enterohepatic recirculation)	Feces and urine	• Severe sinus node dysfunction • Advanced heart block without pacemaker • Symptomatic bradycardia • Cardiogenic shock • Severe liver dysfunction • Severe thyroid dysfunction	• Hypotension(IV) • Photosensitivity • Abnormal gait • Impaired memory • Fatigue and dizziness • Elevated liver enzymes • Visual disturbances • Hypothyroidism
Dronedarone						
• Atrial fibrillation • Atrial flutter	3-6 hours	13-19 hours	Hepatic	Feces and urine	• Permanent Afib • Symptomatic heart failure • Advanced heart block without a pacemaker • Significant bradycardia • Prolonged QT interval(>500ms)	• Prolonged QTc • Increased serum Creatinine • Bradycardia • Diarrhea, nausea and vomiting • Weakness
Sotalol						
• Sustained ventricular tachycardia • Maintenance of sinus rhythm	1-2 hours (oral) 5 to 10 min (IV)	12 hours	none	Urine	• Bronchial asthma • Severe bradycardia • Heart block without a pacemaker • Long QT syndrome • Decompensated heart failure • cardiogenic shock	• Bradycardia • Chest pain and palpitation • Weakness • Dyspnea • Edema • Nausea and vomiting
Ibutilide						
• Acute termination of atrial fibrillation or flutter • Pretreatment for electrical cardioversion	90 Min (only IV)	2-12 hrs	Extensive hepatic	Urine and feces	• QTc >440ms in presence of bradycardia, hypokalemia and QT prolonging drugs	• Ventricular tachycardia • Headache • Nausea and vomiting • Q-T prolongation
Dofetilide						
• Conversion of atrial fibrillation in flutter • Maintenance sinus rhythm after cardioversion of atrial fibrillation	2-3 hours	10 hours	Hepatic	Urine	• Long QT syndrome • QTc >440 Sec (>500 sec in BBB) • Severe renal impairment • Concurrent use of QT prolonging drugs	• Headache • Dizziness • Ventricular tachycardia • Chest pain • Torsade de Pointes (within 3 days of initiation)

Table 13.4 Class III antiarrhythmics

is primarily cleared through the kidney.

Class IV Antiarrhythmics

These agents are otherwise known as **Calcium channel blockers**. Depending on the chemical properties and resulting pharmacodynamic effect, Calcium channel blockers are classified into **Dihydropyridines** (**Nifedi**_pine_, **Amlodi**_pine_, **Felodi**_pine_, **Nicardi**_pine_ etc.) and **non-dihydropyridines** (**Verapamil** and **Diltiazem**). Because of the predominant inhibitory effect on SA and AV node, *non-dihydropyridines have pertinent electrophysiologic properties* compared to that of dihydropyridines. **Verapamil** and **Diltiazem** are commonly used for *rate control* especially in atrial arrhythmias. These agents *prolong AV node conduction* and *refractoriness* and thereby reduced ventricular rate in AV nodal re-entry tachycardia. They do not have much effect on ventricular arrhythmias. Non-dihydropyridines calcium channel blockers are used for various other purposes in cardiovascular medicine including management of hypertension, vasospastic angina, hypertrophic cardiomyopathy etc.

> **Verapamil** should not be administered intravenously in any patients with a wide complex tachycardia unless it is absolutely certain about the type of rhythm and the response of the patient to Verapamil in that setting.

Influence of non-dihydropyridine calcium channel blockers on AV node is more pronounced during faster heart rate (**use dependent channel block**). It increases refractoriness of both antegrade and retrograde conduction pathway in the AV node. Therefore, these agents are particularly *useful for rate control in nodal re-entry tachycardia*. **Verapamil** *does not affect the refractoriness of accessory pathways*. Intravenous administration of Verapamil during atrial fibrillation in patients with WPW syndrome can precipitate ventricular tachycardia through accessory conduction.

Non-dihydropyridine calcium channel blockers generally cause *peripheral vasodilatation and in higher doses can cause myocardial suppression*. They can also cause orthostatic hypotension, bradycardia and atrio ventricular block. Non-dihydropyridine calcium channel blockers are contraindicated in patients with advanced heart failure, second or third degree heart block without a pacemaker, WPW syndrome, wide complex tachycardia, cardiogenic shock, severe aortic stenosis etc.

When used together with Digoxin, Verapamil can reduce excretion of Digoxin and thereby increasing Digoxin effect. In the event of Digoxin toxicity, concomitant use of Verapamil can cause complete heart block. Overdose with calcium channel blockers can be treated with administration of **Calcium gluconate**.For detailed description of Calcium channel blockers, please refer chapter 4.

Class V Antiarrhythmics

Digoxin and **Adenosine** are categorized in this group of antiarrhythmics. Among these, Digoxin implies it is antiarrhythmic properties due to *increased vagal tone* and thereby reducing rate of sinus node discharge and prolongs AV node refractoriness. It has *minimal effect on the ventricles and the bundle branch system*. The peak effect of intravenously administered Digoxin can be seen within three hours and oral dosing in six hours. Since it is excreted through the kidney, the dosage of Digoxin should be adjusted for patients with renal dysfunction.

Digoxin produces *increasing contractility* (*positive ionotropic effect*) in myocardium by *increasing intracellular Calcium* concentration. Because of the smaller therapeutic window (**0.8** - **1.2** ng/ml), Digoxin needs *frequent monitoring of blood levels*. It also interacts with many other drugs including Amiodarone, Warfarin etc. In toxic dosage, Digoxin cause *high-grade atrioventricular block* or *accelerated junctional rhythm* and at times *ventricular tachycardia*.

> Since **Digoxin** acts through ***vagal mechanism***, effect of Digoxin is largely unnoticed during exercise and activity. Therefore, ambulatory patients should be treated with a combination of Beta blockers and Digoxin to prevent exercise induced rapid ventricular response.

Because of the slow pharmacologic action of Digoxin compared to that of Adenosine and other non-dihydropyridine calcium channel blockers, it is *not used for acute termination of tachyarrhythmia*. However, Digoxin is very useful in *ventricular rate control for chronic atrial fibrillation*.

In patients with **WPW pattern** of EKG, Digoxin administration should be avoided because of the risk of *delaying AV nodal conduction and promoting accessory pathway*, leading to *ventricular tachyarrhythmia*. Symptoms of Digoxin toxicity include headache, nausea and vomiting, altered color perception, generalized weakness etc. At toxic levels, Digoxin can cause sinus bradycardia, sinus arrest, junctional rhythms etc. Patients with impaired renal function, advanced age, hypokalemia, hypothyroidism and chronic lung disease are more susceptible for Digoxin toxicity. **Digoxin immune FAB** antibody therapy can be used in severe Digoxin toxicity. *Tachyarrhythmia secondary to Digoxin toxicity should not be treated with DC cardioversion* because of the risk of life-threatening ventricular tachycardia or ventricular fibrillation.

Class V Antiarrhythmics

Indication	Onset/ Peak	Half-life	Metabolism	Elimination	Contraindication	Side-effects
Digoxin						
• Rate control in atrial fibrillation • Class II to III heart failure	1-2 hours (Oral) 5-60 min (IV)	36-48 hours	Stomach and intestine	Urine	• Ventricular fibrillation • Hypersensitivity to digoxin	• Accelerated junctional rhythm • Atrial tachycardia with or without block • Heart block • PVC, VT, V fib
Adenosine						
• Paroxysmal SVT	Rapid	<10 sec	Blood and tissue	None	• Second or third degree heart block • Sick sinus syndrome • Severe bradycardia	• Hypotension • New onset arrhythmia (Transient) • GI discomfort • Headache, chest pressure, dyspnea • Discomfort at neck, jaw and throat

Table 13.5 Class V antiarrythmic agents

Adenosine acts through specialized *potassium channels* within the atrium, SA and AV node. Because of the lack of these channels in ventricular myocardium, Adenosine *does not have any direct effect on ventricles*. Rapid intravenous injection of Adenosine produces profound and transient AV nodal conduction block and therefore useful in termination of **paroxysmal SVT**. Adenosine is useful in *differentiating supraventricular tachycardia with aberrancy* from that of *ventricular tachycardia* as it can terminate most of SVT however, does not affect arrhythmia from ventricular origin.

If the patient has concomitant use of **Theophylline**, *Adenosine does not work* because of Adenosine receptor blockade from Theophylline. Due to the possible micro re-entry circuit within the atria, Adenosine can produce *atrial fibrillation in 10-15% of patients*. Use of **Dipyridamole** can prolong the effect of Adenosine and therefore should be used with caution. Because of

Major Therapeutic Use of Antiarrhythmic Agents*

Drug Class		SVT	Atrial fib	Atrial flutter	AVNRT	WPW	PVC	VT
Class I A	Quinidine	•	•	•			•	
	Procainamide		•			•		•
	Disopyramide		•					•
Class I B	Lidocaine							•
	Mexiletine						•	•
Class I C	Flecainide	•	•					•
	Propafenone	•	•					
Class II		•	•	•			•	
Class III	Amiodarone	•	•		•			•
	Dronedarone		•	•				
	Sotalol		•					•
	Ibutilide		•	•				
	Dofetilide		•					
Class IV	Verapamil**		•	•	•			
	Diltiazem**		•	•	•			
Class V	Digoxin		•					
	Adenosine	•						

* Only major indications are represented. ; ** Mainly for rate control

Table 13.6. Major therapeutic use of antiarrhythmic agents

the short duration of action and increased effectiveness, *Adenosine is preferred over non-dihydropyridine calcium channel blockers in termination of supraventricular tachycardia,* especially in patients with hypotension, heart failure etc. Adenosine should not be used in patients with active bronchoconstriction as it can worsen respiratory distress. Other transient side effects of chest pressure, dyspnea and flushing that may last less than 1 min can be seen and are well tolerated.

Points to remember!!!

- Electrophysiologic effects of antiarrhythmic agents depend on the type of the tissue, membrane potential, heart rate, genetic variations, age etc.

- Class **I** agents are **sodium channel blockers**, **Beta-blockers** in class **II**, **Potassium channel blockers** in class **III** and **Calcium channel blockers** in class **IV**. Adenosine and Digoxin are classified as class **V.**

- Class I Antiarrhythmic Drugs known as Sodium channel blockers and they control the *movement of sodium ions in phase 0* of cardiac action potential curve.

- Depending on the ease of binding and dissociation with the receptor sites, Class I antiarrhythmics are further classified into class **1C** (having *slowest rate of binding and dissociation*), class **1B** (has *rapid binding and release*) and class **1A** (with *intermediate binding and dissociation*).

- Class **1C** drugs (**Flecainide** and **Propafenone**) when used during fast heart rate, takes more time to dissociate from the receptor sites and make less number of receptors available for active contractile function. This property is called **use dependent channel block**.

- Some drugs exert greater effects at slow heart rate than at the fast rate known as **reverse use dependent channel blockers**.

- The efficacy of sodium channel blocking property is *highest for class 1C drugs, followed by class 1A and class 1B*

- Class 1A Antiarrhythmic Agents (e.g. Quinidine, Procanamide and Disopyramide) have intermediate sodium channel blocking property and can cause **Torsades De Pointes** especially in patients with prolonged base line QT interval and electrolyte abnormalities.

- Only in patients with *pre-existing sinus node dysfunction,* **Quinidine** *depresses sinus node automaticity.*

- Using Quinidine along *with other vasodilators may cause significant hypotension.*

- Quinidine is particularly useful in *treatment of premature supraventricular and ventricular complexes, AV nodal re-entry tachycardia* (AVNRT) and *termination of atrial flutter of atrial fibrillation.*

- Syncope episodes while on Quinidine are mostly because of the Q-T prolongation and are treated with intravenous Magnesium.

- Procainamide exerts its effects through *reducing automaticity, conductivity and excitability of the conduction system* as Quinidine.

- Procainamide has least amount of anticholinergic effects among all the drugs in class **1A** and therefore *is better tolerated than Quinidine.*

- Procainamide is used for treatment of *supraventricular and ventricular arrhythmias, treatment of new onset atrial fibrillation or flutter, atrial fibrillation with WPW syndrome etc.*

- *Atrial fibrillation with rapid ventricular response should be treated with beta or calcium channel blockers prior to the use of Procanamide* in order to avoid ventricular tachyarrhythmia from possible 1:1 conduction through the AV node

- Common side effects from Procanamide treatment are *myalgia, Raynaud's phenomena, agranulocytosis, prolonged QT syndrome* leading to *polymorphic VT.*

- Procanamide may *increase defibrillation threshold.*

- **Disopyramide (Norpace®)** is used for treatment of *recurrent ventricular tachycardia and atrial fibrillation.*

- Disopyramide can cause *Q-T prolongation and polymorphic*

VT along with less serious side effects like urinary retention, constipation, dry mouth etc.

- **Lidocaine** and **Mexiletine** are classified into class **1B** antiarrhythmics and are particularly *useful in treating ventricular arrhythmias* in the setting of myocardial infarction
- **Lidocaine** has *rapid onset and offset from its receptors* and has extensive **first pass metabolism.**
- **Mexiletine** is useful for oral treatment of patients with *symptomatic ventricular tachycardia*.
- **Class 1C Antiarrhythmic Agents (Flecainide** and **Propafenone)** are used for treatment of *atrial fibrillation*.
- Flecainide and Propafenone can cause harmful effects in patients *with structural heart disease* such as prior history of myocardium ischemia or infarction and are generally *contraindicated*.
- Because of the slow dissociation of Flecainide from sodium channels, significant effect of this drug is seen in lower heart rates (**reverse use dependence**).
- Flecainide is useful for treatment of *non-sustained ventricular tachycardia, atrial tachycardia, flutter* and *fibrillation*.
- Most important adverse effects of Flecainide is its *pro arrhythmic effect* and is seen in up to 30% of patients especially *with underlying cardiac decompensation* and *ventricular arrhythmia*.
- **Propafenone** is used for treatment of *paroxysmal supraventricular tachycardia, atrial fibrillation, non-sustained and sustained ventricular tachycardia*.
- Propafenone is used with *caution in patients having severe left ventricular dysfunction* because of the negative ionotropic property; however, has a better side effect profile than Flecainide.
- Class II Antiarrhythmics are otherwise known as Beta-blockers, with their characteristic beta-adrenergic receptor blockade property and thereby *suppression of arrhythmias resulting from*

autonomic nervous system stimulation.

- Beta-blockers can be **selective beta I receptor blockers** (cardio selective) or **non-selective beta blockers** (non-cardio selective).

- Beta-blockers are particularly useful in controlling arrhythmias associated with high catecholamine states such as *thyrotoxicosis, pheochromocytoma* or those related with adrenergic stimulation from *exercise, emotions* or use of stimulants like *cocaine*.

- Class III Antiarrhythmics have characteristic potassium channel blocking properties.

- They cause *increase in duration of cardiac action potential* and therefore *prolong QT interval* in EKG.

- Amiodarone shows more of *class I* and *IV properties* (*sodium* and *calcium channel blocking*) and thereby effectively *treats faster ventricular arrhythmias when given intravenously during an acute myocardial event.*

- When given *intravenously compared to oral route, Amiodarone can cause negative ionotropic effect* in the left ventricle

- Amiodarone is used for treatment of supraventricular and ventricular arrhythmias including *re-entry tachycardia, atrial flutter* and *fibrillation, ventricular tachycardia* or *fibrillation*.

- Amiodarone can *reduce the incidence of spontaneous ventricular tachycardia* and resultant shock therapy in patients with implantable cardioverter defibrillator (ICD).

- Long term Amiodarone use can create side effects like *chronic interstitial pneumonitis, thyroid dysfunction, photosensitivity, peripheral neuropathy* etc.

- Amiodarone has shown to increase **defibrillation threshold** (energy required for successful conversion of ventricular tachyarrhythmia).

- Dronedarone is indicated for *chemical cardioversion of atrial fibrillation or flutter* and *maintenance of sinus rhythm after conversion*.

- Dronedarone is slightly less effective than Amiodarone however, because of the lack of iodine molecule; has a better side effect profile

- Dronedarone is *contraindicated for use in patients with underlying advanced heart failure.*
- **Sotalol** is a nonselective beta-blocker without intrinsic sympathomimetic activity and is useful in treatment of *ventricular arrhythmias, atrial fibrillation* and other *supraventricular tachycardia.*
- Side effects of sotalol include *bradycardia* that is due to beta blocking property and *Q-T prolongation* and *risk of polymorphic VT*
- Unlike Amiodarone, *Sotalol reduces the defibrillation threshold.*
- Because of predominant renal clearance, Sotalol is *not ideal in renal dysfunction.* I
- Ibutilide is a class III potassium channel blocker administered intravenously and is used for *acute termination of established atrial fibrillation or flutter.*
- Serious side effects of Ibutilide is the incidence of *Q-T prolongation and Torsades de Pointes*
- **Dofetilide (Tikosyn®)** is an oral class **III** antiarrhythmic agent used for both *conversion of atrial fibrillation* and *termination of recurrent episodes* of atrial fibrillation in long-term.
- *High incidence of Q-T prolongation and resultant Torsades de Pointes* is seen as a complication of Dofetilide.
- Class IV Antiarrhythmics (Calcium channel blockers) are classified into Dihydropyridines (Nifedipine, Amlodipine, Felodipine, Nicardipine etc.) and non-dihydropyridines (Verapamil and Diltiazem).
- Because of the predominant inhibitory effect on SA and AV node, *non-dihydropyridines have pertinent electrophysiologic properties* compared to that of dihydropyridines.
- **Verapamil** *does not affect the refractoriness of accessory pathways* and therefore, intravenous administration of

Verapamil during atrial fibrillation in patients with WPW syndrome can precipitate ventricular tachycardia

- Non-dihydropyridine calcium channel blockers generally cause *peripheral vasodilatation and in higher doses can cause myocardial suppression.*
- Overdose with calcium channel blockers can be treated with administration of **Calcium gluconate**.
- **Digoxin** and **Adenosine** are categorized as Class V antiarrhythmics.
- Digoxin implies it is antiarrhythmic properties due to *increased vagal tone* and thereby reducing rate of sinus node discharge and prolongs AV node refractoriness. It has *minimal effect on the ventricles and the bundle branch system.*
- Digoxin produces *increasing contractility* (*positive ionotropic effect*) in myocardium by *increasing intracellular Calcium* concentration.
- Because of the smaller therapeutic window (**0.8** - **1.2** ng/ml), Digoxin needs *frequent monitoring of blood levels.*
- Digoxin cause *high-grade atrioventricular block* or *accelerated junctional rhythm* and at times *ventricular tachycardia* in toxic serum concentration.
- *Digoxin is not used for acute termination of tachyarrhythmia Because of the slow pharmacologic action.*
- **WPW pattern** of EKG, Digoxin administration should be avoided because of the risk of *delaying AV nodal conduction and promoting accessory pathway*; leading to *ventricular tachyarrhythmia.*
- *Tachyarrhythmia secondary to Digoxin toxicity should not be treated with DC cardioversion* because of the risk of life-threatening ventricular tachycardia or ventricular fibrillation.
- **Adenosine** acts through specialized *potassium channels* within the atrium, SA and AV node.
- Adenosine *does not have any direct effect on ventricles.*

- Rapid intravenous injection of Adenosine produce profound and transient AV nodal conduction block and therefore useful in termination of **paroxysmal SVT**.

- If the patient has concomitant use of **Theophylline**, *Adenosine does not work* because of Adenosine receptor blockade from Theophylline.

Index

A

B

E

F

G

H

I

J

K

L

M

Q

R

S

T

U

V

W

X

Z

76260265R00104

Made in the USA
Columbia, SC
23 September 2019